NEONATAL SKIN CARE

EVIDENCE-BASED CLINICAL PRACTICE GUIDELINE

3rd Edition

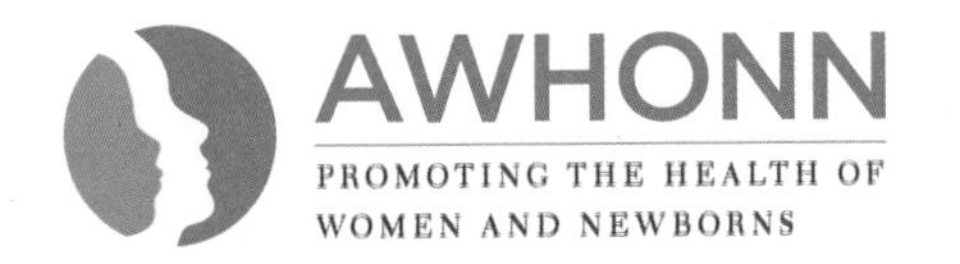

Association of Women's Health, Obstetric and Neonatal Nurses

The Association of Women's Health, Obstetric and Neonatal Nurses (AWHONN) is accredited as a provider of continuing nursing education by the American Nurses Credentialing Center's (ANCC's) Commission on Accreditation.

Accredited status does not imply endorsement by AWHONN or ANCC of any commercial products displayed or discussed in conjunction with this activity.

AWHONN requires authors, reviewers, and nurse planners in a position to control content of continuing nursing education resources to disclose all relevant financial relationships with any commercial interest.

Guideline Development Science Team:

- Carolyn Houska Lund is a member of the Johnson & Johnson Scientific Advisory Board and a member of the 3M Scientific Advisory Board. She is a co-investigator for an investigator-initiated study supported by Johnson & Johnson about how the newborn's first bath affects skin parameters and the bacterial microbiome of the skin.
- Debra Brandon reports no relevant financial relationships with commercial interests
- Catherine M. Hill reports no relevant financial relationships with commercial interests.
- Ann C. Holden reports no relevant financial relationships with commercial interests.
- Joanne Kuller is a co-investigator for an investigator-initiated study supported by Johnson & Johnson about how the newborn's first bath affects skin parameters and the bacterial microbiome of the skin.

Reviewers:

- Janet Pettit was paid an honorarium by Professional Disposables International, which manufactures skin disinfectant agents, for a presentation in October 2012.
- Janice M. Thape reports no relevant financial relationships with commercial interests.
- Dr. Albert Yan reports no relevant financial relationships with commercial interests.

Nurse Planner/Reviewer:

Anne Santa-Donato, the nurse planner, reports no relevant financial relationships with commercial interests. The nurse planner has mitigated the risk of commercial bias by participating in the review of this Evidence-Based Clinical Practice Guideline throughout the development process and by developing its associated continuing education activity with the project manager. All members of the science team, the project manager and reviewers are charged with the responsibility to ensure that the content of the guideline and the continuing nursing education activity is free of commercial bias.

This Evidence-Based Clinical Practice Guideline was developed for AWHONN, as an informational resource for nursing practice. The Guideline does not define a standard of care, nor is it intended to dictate an exclusive course of management. It presents general methods and techniques of practice that AWHONN believes to be currently and widely viewed as acceptable, based on current research and recognized authorities.

Proper care of individual patients may depend on many individual factors to be considered in clinical practice, as well as professional judgment in the techniques described herein. Variations and innovations that are consistent with law and that demonstrably improve the quality of patient care should be encouraged. AWHONN believes the drug classifications and selections set forth in this text are in accordance with current recommendations and practice at the time of publication. However, in view of ongoing research, changes in government regulations, and the constant flow of information relating to drug therapy and drug reactions, the reader is urged to check information available in other published sources for each drug for potential changes in indications, dosages, warnings, and precautions. This is particularly important when a recommended agent is a new or infrequently employed drug. In addition, appropriate medication use may depend on unique factors such as individuals' health status, other medication use, and other factors that the professional must consider in clinical practice.

The information presented here is not designed to define standards of practice for employment, licensure, discipline, legal, or other purposes.

ACKNOWLEDGEMENTS
Neonatal Skin Care

The Neonatal Skin Care Evidence-Based Clinical Practice Guideline and Quick Care Guide were developed by the Evidence-Based Clinical Practice Guideline Development Team, which is comprised of member experts of both AWHONN and the National Association of Neonatal Nurses (NANN) who are nationally recognized for their significant contributions in neonatal nursing. The team members were selected for this revision by AWHONN for their expertise as scientists and clinicians dedicated to improving the health and well-being of women and newborns.

The process for Guideline development described herein was the result of the combined efforts of AWHONN's Practice, Research and Education committees undertaken in 1998 using the framework presented in the American Nurses Association (ANA) *Manual to Develop Guidelines* (Marek, 1995). AWHONN gratefully acknowledges the work of the individuals who have contributed their time and expertise to promoting evidence-based practice in nursing and who have been instrumental in disseminating a growing body of knowledge about neonatal skin care.

AWHONN acknowledges and appreciates the contributions of the AWHONN and NANN members who participated in development and revision of the first and second editions of this Guideline.

2011–2013 NEONATAL SKIN CARE EVIDENCE-BASED CLINICAL PRACTICE GUIDELINE DEVELOPMENT SCIENCE TEAM

Carolyn Houska Lund, MS, RN, FAAN, Team Leader

Debra Brandon, PhD, RN, CCNS, FAAN

Ann C. Holden, BScN, MScT, RN

Joanne Kuller, RN, MS, NANN Representative

Catherine M. Hill, MSN, FNP-BC, Project Manager

REVIEWERS

Debra Bingham, DrPH, RN

Janet Pettit, DNP, NNP-BC, VA-BC, CNS

Janice M. Thape, MSN, RNC-NIC, CWONc

Albert Yan, MD, FAAP, FAAD

Anne Santa-Donato, MSN, RNC, Nurse Planner

TABLE OF CONTENTS

Neonatal Skin Care

EVIDENCE-BASED CLINICAL PRACTICE GUIDELINE DEVELOPMENT

Scope of the Evidence-Based Clinical Practice Guideline

PURPOSE STATEMENT

The purpose of this Guideline is to provide registered nurses (RNs) and advanced practice registered nurses (APRNs) with clinical practice recommendations for neonatal skin care based on the best available evidence. The goal is to optimize neonatal skin integrity through the provision of nursing care based on scientific principles and empiric evidence. This Guideline describes evidence-based approaches to accomplish the following:

- Assess the neonate's skin condition.
- Identify neonates who are or may be at risk for alterations in skin integrity.
- Recognize environmental and treatment-related agents that may alter neonatal skin integrity.
- Implement interventions to promote and protect optimal skin function for low-and high-risk neonates.
- Support normal skin development.
- Minimize the potential for future skin sensitization.

PATIENT POPULATION

The Guideline is directed toward neonates (birth to 28 days of age) of all gestational ages. The only exclusion criteria are neonates with congenital skin disorders. Elements of the Guideline are applicable for healthy as well as high-risk and sick neonates.

SETTINGS

The Guideline is applicable in all neonatal health care settings and other health care facilities that provide care during the post-birth neonatal period, such as freestanding birthing centers. Relevant components of the Guideline may be applicable in the home setting.

PROVIDERS

The Guideline is directed toward RNs and APRNs responsible for managing or providing care to neonates. Other licensed or unlicensed personnel accountable to the RN or APRN may use the Guideline as appropriate for their level of responsibility for patient care and within the scope of clinical practice defined by licensing boards or accrediting bodies. Selected elements of the Guideline may be appropriate for use by parents or other caregivers when a neonate is discharged to the home before 28 days of age.

EVIDENCE-BASED CLINICAL PRACTICE GUIDELINE ELEMENTS

Using the original Neonatal Skin Care Evidence-Based Clinical Practice Guideline as a template, the Guideline development team reviewed and scored relevant literature according to the process described below. Team members were then assigned to revise the following individual elements of the Evidence-Based Clinical Practice Guideline:

- Newborn skin assessment
- Bathing, including first bath, routine bathing, and immersion bathing
- Vernix caseosa
- Umbilical cord care
- Circumcision care
- Disinfectants

- Diaper dermatitis and diaper wipes
- Medical adhesives
- Emollients
- Transepidermal water loss (TEWL)
- Skin breakdown
- Intravenous (IV) extravasation

Through weekly teleconferences, team members reviewed each of the above elements and achieved consensus on each clinical practice recommendation, accompanying referenced rationale, and quality-of-evidence rating.

EVIDENCE–BASED GUIDELINE DEVELOPMENT PROCESS

The use of research findings to guide and evaluate clinical practice has a profound impact on the nursing process and the quality of care provided to women around the world (Scott, 2010). Nursing specialty organizations are in a unique position to facilitate the use of research findings in clinical practice through the guideline development process.

AWHONN is known as a leader among nursing organizations in the international movement to develop guidelines for evidence-based decision-making in accordance with its mission to improve the health of women and newborns. The original AWHONN template for guideline development is based on the framework delineated in the ANA *Manual to Develop Guidelines* (Marek, 1995). The ANA *Manual* models its process on that of the Agency for Healthcare Research and Quality, formerly the Agency for Health Care Policy and Research (Woolf, 1990, 1992).

Development of the first edition of the Neonatal Skin Care Evidence-Based Clinical Practice Guideline began in 2000 following completion of the original AWHONN/NANN Neonatal Skin Care Research-Based Practice Project (known as RBP4). The first- and second-edition Evidence-Based Clinical Practice Guideline development teams were comprised of members of the original RBP4 science team and selected site coordinators. New members were added for both the second and third editions as needed to replace original team members. The Evidence-Based Clinical Practice Guideline development science team for the third edition convened in the fall of 2011. Content from the second edition of the Guideline was updated and revised to include new information about newborn skin physiology and atopic dermatitis.

For the third edition of this Guideline, topic-specific searches of several electronic databases and manual searches were conducted to identify relevant literature. Specifically, MEDLINE, the Cumulative Index to Nursing and Allied Health Literature (CINAHL), PubMed, and the Cochrane Library were searched for journal articles written in English and published between 2007 and 2012. Articles reporting the results of a variety of clinical trials, review articles, and reports of case studies were reviewed and scored. Duplicate citations were identified and eliminated.

The primary search term used was *neonatal skin care* with the inclusion of subcategories of *skin assessment, newborn bathing, immersion bathing, umbilical cord care, circumcision care, intravenous infiltration, skin breakdown, diaper dermatitis, diaper wipes, atopic dermatitis, transepidermal water loss, products, sunscreens, microbiome, microbiology and skin development, adhesives, emollients, disinfectants, and vernix caseosa.* Additional articles, including selected articles published before 2007 and after the original literature search was completed in 2012, were retrieved and scored based on knowledge of seminal works and as new topics or as gaps in the literature were identified. A total of 332 articles were reviewed and scored by the science team for inclusion as supporting rationale for clinical practice recommendations in the guideline.

Literature Evaluation and Scoring

A system and tool for scoring the quantitative literature was developed based on the method for literature analysis presented in the ANA *Manual* (Marek, 1995). Using this framework, each study reviewed by the Guideline team was evaluated using the following eight criteria:

- Problem or question studied: Clearly stated, significant, and relevant problem
- Sampling: Representative sampling, less than 20% dropout rate, and random selection process
- Measurement: Tools/methods appropriate, reliable, and valid
- Internal validity: Accurate conclusions about covariation
- External validity: Valid conclusions about generalizability
- Construct validity: Appropriate independent and dependent variables identified
- Statistical conclusion validity: Statistical significance supported by data ($p \leq 0.05$)
- Justification for conclusions: Causal conclusions justified

A description of the above criteria and a sample scoring tool can be found in the ANA *Manual* (Marek, 1995).

Quality-of-Evidence Rating

As the Evidence-Based Clinical Practice Guideline was further developed, the quality of quantitative evidence supporting clinical practice recommendations was determined by team consensus using the U.S. Preventive Services Task Force (1996) Guide to Clinical Preventive Services quality-of-evidence rating scale:

I: Evidence obtained from at least one properly designed randomized, controlled trial or metaanalysis of randomized, controlled trials.

II-1: Evidence obtained from well-designed controlled trials without randomization.

II-2: Evidence obtained from well-designed cohort or case–control analytic studies, preferably from more than one center or research group.

II-3: Evidence from multiple time series with or without the intervention. Dramatic results in uncontrolled experiments (such as the results of the introduction of penicillin treatment in the 1940s) could also be regarded as this type of evidence.

III: Opinions of respected authorities, based on clinical experience, descriptive studies, or reports of expert committees.

INSTRUCTIONS FOR COMPLETING THE CONTINUING NURSING EDUCATION (CNE) ACTIVITY

This Evidence-Based Clinical Practice Guideline includes an optional CNE activity. Upon successful completion of this activity, the participant will be able to:

- assess the neonate's skin condition,
- support normal neonatal skin development,
- identify neonates who may be at risk for alterations in skin integrity,
- recognize environmental and treatment-related agents that may alter skin integrity,
- implement interventions to promote and protect optimal skin function, and
- minimize the potential for future skin sensitization.

Effective with the date of publication of this Guideline, **2.8** contact hours are available for successful completion of the CNE activity until **December 31, 2015**. To successfully complete the CNE activity, the participant must read the entire Guideline, purchase and complete the CNE Companion for Neonatal Skin Care: Evidence-Based Clinical Practice Guideline, 3rd Edition, which includes a posttest and CNE participant feedback form. Additional details about obtaining CNE contact hours are provided in Appendix D.

Evolving Concepts in Neonatal Skin Care

OVERVIEW OF NEONATAL SKIN AND SKIN CARE PRACTICES

Neonatal skin and skin care is an important clinical concern for nurses who care for newborns, including well, full-term, healthy premature, and extremely premature neonates. High value is also placed on using evidence-based practices for newborns. In 2001, AWHONN and NANN published the first edition of *Neonatal Skin Care Evidence-Based Clinical Practice Guidelines*, one of the first such documents of its kind for neonatal skin care (AWHONN, 2001). Subsequently, the use of this Guideline was evaluated in 51 nurseries in the United States, and improvements in neonatal skin condition and positive changes in clinical practice were demonstrated (Lund, Kuller, Lane, et al., 2001; Lund, Osborne, Kuller, et al., 2001). The second edition of the Guideline was published in 2007, incorporating current research and evidence for practice changes (AWHONN 2007). The third edition of the guideline has been updated to include current evidence-based clinical practice recommendations for newborn skin care based on the review of the literature described previously.

PHYSIOLOGIC AND ANATOMIC VARIATIONS IN TERM NEWBORN AND PREMATURE INFANT SKIN

Understanding the unique physiologic and anatomic differences in neonatal and premature infant skin (compared with the skin of adults) is fundamental to evaluating and integrating new information into neonatal skin care practices. Newborn skin undergoes an adaptation process during the transition from the aquatic environment of the uterus to the aerobic environment after birth. The skin assists in thermoregulation, serves as a barrier against toxins and microorganisms, is a reservoir for fat storage and insulation, and is a primary interface for tactile sensation and communication with the mother (Lund & Kuller, 2007).

The skin of the full-term newborn is coated with vernix caseosa, a cheese-like substance that contains sebum from sebaceous glands, broken-off lanugo and desquamated cells from the amnion, as well as water. Vernix begins to form as early as 17–20 weeks of gestation, with the thickest coating noted between 36 and 38 weeks. By 40 weeks, it is found primarily in skin creases. Vernix protects the fetus from maceration from amniotic fluid and allows the fetus to move without chafing as it grows in utero. Vernix caseosa assists in the development of the "acid mantle" of the skin surface, which inhibits the growth of pathogenic microorganisms and imparts immunologic properties to the skin (Larson & Dinulos, 2005; Tollin et al., 2005).

Premature infant skin is thinner than the skin of full-term newborns and typically looks transparent, even gelatinous, in the most immature infants. The skin may appear "ruddy" because the blood vessels are closer to the surface, and there are fewer wrinkles. These vulnerabilities pose significant challenges to maintaining skin integrity for the premature infant.

Stratum Corneum and Epidermis

The stratum corneum, which provides the important barrier function of the skin, contains 10–20 layers in both adults and full-term newborns. Although full-term newborn skin has been shown to have skin barrier function comparable to adult skin when measured using TEWL assessment techniques (Yosipovitch, Maayan-Metzger, Merlob, & Sirota, 2000), more recent evidence has revealed that the stratum corneum does not function as well as adult skin throughout the first year of life and is approximately 30% thinner than that of adult skin (Nikolovski, Stamatas, Kollias, & Wiegand, 2008). The basal layer of the epidermis, directly underneath the stratum corneum, is approximately 20% thinner than that of the adult, and the keratinocyte cells in this layer have a higher cell turnover rate, which may account for the faster wound healing that has been observed in neonates (Stamatas, Nikolovski, Mack, & Kollias, 2011).

The premature infant has far fewer layers of stratum corneum compared with the full-term newborn, depending on gestational age. At less than 30 weeks of gestation, there may be as few as two or three layers (Holbrook, 1982), and the extremely premature infant of 23–24 weeks has negligible barrier function due to minimal stratum corneum (Agren, Sjors, & Sedin, 1998). The deficiency of the stratum corneum results in large fluid and evaporative heat losses in the first weeks of life, which can lead to significant alterations in electrolyte levels, hypernatremia, and dehydration (Bhatia, 2006). Techniques used to reduce these losses include the application of polyethylene coverings immediately after birth (Bissinger & Annibale, 2010; Knobel, Simmer, & Holbert, 2005; Vohra, Roberts, Zhang, Janes, & Schmidt, 2004) and use of high humidity environments in incubators (Gaylord, Wright, Lorch, Lorch, & Walker, 2001; Kim, Lee, Chen, & Ringer, 2010). Topical treatments such as the application of transparent adhesive dressings (Bhandari, Brodsky, & Porat, 2005; Mancini, Sookdeo-Drost, Madison, Smoller, & Lane, 1994) and sterile topical ointment and skin protectants have been described in small studies (Beeram, Olvera, Krauss, Loughran, & Petty, 2006; Brandon, Coe, Hudson-Barr, Oliver, & Landerman, 2010), but these treatments remain the subject of debate due to concerns about infection.

Maturation of the stratum corneum in premature infants was once thought to occur in the first 14 days after birth, as a result of the impact of the atmosphere and influx of water (Harpin & Rutter, 1983). Other studies show a slower process of maturation, particularly for infants of 23–25 weeks of gestation (Agren et al., 1998; Sedin, Hammarlund, Nilsson, Stromberg, & Oberg, 1985), who have impaired barrier function until they reach 30–32 weeks' postconceptional age (Kalia, Nonato, Lund, & Guy, 1998).

Dermis and the Cohesion between Epidermis and Dermis

The dermis in the newborn is thinner and not as well developed as the adult dermis. Collagen fibers are shorter and less dense, and the reticular layer of the dermis is absent, which makes the skin feel soft. There is also less total lipid and fewer sebaceous glands compared with adult skin glands (Stamatas, Nikolovski, et al., 2011).

Between the epidermis and dermis are fibrils that connect these two layers of the skin. In premature infants, the fibrils are fewer in number than in full-term or adult epidermis, with wide spaces between connecting points (Holbrook, 1982). As the premature infant matures, these fibrils increase in number and strength.

The decreased cohesion between the epidermis and dermis places the premature newborn at risk for skin injury when medical adhesives attached to the skin are removed. When extremely strong adhesives are used, the bond between the adhesive and the epidermis may be stronger than that between the epidermis and dermis, resulting in stripping of the epidermal layer and decreased skin barrier function (Lund & Kuller, 2007).

Skin pH

Full-term newborns are born with an alkaline skin surface (pH > 6.0), but within 96 hours of life, the pH typically falls to less than 5.0 (Behrendt & Green, 1971). In a study comparing full-term newborns with adults, the mean pH of the newborn skin measured 7.08 on the first day of life, while the adult skin pH was 5.7 (Yosipovitch et al., 2000). The retention of vernix caseosa has been shown to assist in the development of the acid mantle in newborn skin (Visscher et al., 2005).

The skin surface pH in premature infants of varying gestational ages has been reported to be more than 6 on the first day of life, decreasing to 5.5 by the end of the first week, and then to 5.1 by the end of the first month of life (Fox, Nelson, & Wareham 1998). Bathing and other topical treatments transiently affect the skin pH (Gfatter, Hackl, & Braun, 1997), and diapered skin has a higher pH because of the combined effects of urine contact and occlusion (Visscher, Chatterjee, Ebel, LaRuffa, & Hoath, 2002).

Skin Microbiome

In addition to the growing body of knowledge about the unique anatomy and physiology of neonatal skin, recent advances in science and technology have enabled researchers and clinicians to further understand the processes involved in colonization of skin with microorganisms.

Before genetic sequencing for microorganisms was available, microorganisms on and in the human body were identified by cultures, which were sent to a microbiology laboratory and grown to identify the species of microorganism. New molecular technologies, developed as a result of the NIH-sponsored Human Microbiome Project, are now able to detect bacteria that cannot be grown with standard cultures through DNA analysis (Turnbaugh et al., 2007). It is now known that many more species of bacteria exist in and on the human body than were previously thought. Most of these are healthy or commensal bacteria, and some are pathogens. Emerging research has revealed that the number of bacterial cells that live within our bodies exceeds the number of human cells by an estimated factor of 10 and that many of these cells are helpful to the human host (Gregory, 2011; Johnson & Versalovic, 2012; Turnbaugh et al., 2007). The term microbiome describes the collective genomes and gene products of the resident microbes living within and on humans.

In the newborn period and in infancy, the skin microbiome, and possibly the microbiome of the intestinal tract, is influenced by the mode of delivery. For example, the skin is colonized differently in babies born vaginally compared with those delivered by cesarean (Dominguez-Bello, et al, 2010). This difference may have consequences for colonization during the neonatal period with certain pathogens, such as methicillin–resistant *Staphylococcus aureus* (MRSA). In later infancy, the difference in the skin microbiome between babies born vaginally and those born by cesarean may disappear (Capone, Dowd, Stamatas, & Nikolovski, 2011). However, infant skin has different proportions of certain bacterial species than adult skin. The relevance of the influence of mode of delivery on the skin microbiome is not yet clearly understood, but this information has potential for generating a better understanding of how some skin disorders develop and may ultimately assist clinicians in understanding optimal care for skin across the lifespan, including for newborns and infants.

Atopic and Allergic Dermatitis

Among the skin disorders seen in early infancy, atopic dermatitis (also known as eczema) appears to be rising in prevalence, especially in developed countries. The incidence of atopic dermatitis in children has been cited as 20%. Concerns about atopic dermatitis include the association with other atopic diseases, such as asthma and food allergies; this association has been called "the atopic march" as the cascade of symptoms increases (Nicol, 2011).

In infants, atopic dermatitis usually begins on the cheeks, forehead, or scalp and tends to be symmetrically scaly and erythematous. The presence of pruritus is an important aspect of atopic dermatitis and often distinguishes it from other types of rashes. The stratum corneum is compromised in infants with atopic dermatitis; measurements of the stratum corneum hydration are decreased, and TEWL is increased (Nicol, 2011).

Although the etiology of atopic dermatitis is multifactorial, mutations of the filaggrin gene, located in the epidermis, have been identified as a significant predisposing factor (Cork et al., 2006). The sensitization of the newborn skin to allergens may also contribute to the development of atopic dermatitis or result from the impaired barrier function of the stratum corneum of children with atopic dermatitis (Chan, 2008). A pilot study to examine the role of daily moisturization with emollients found a potential protective effect of their use to help prevent atopic dermatitis, and identified the need for a larger trial to determine whether atopic dermatitis can be prevented by improving the skin barrier function in infants with a strong family history of this disorder (Simpson, Berry, Brown, & Hanifin, 2010).

Highlights of the Third Edition

Selected key updates in this edition of the *Neonatal Skin Care Evidence-Based Clinical Practice Guideline* are summarized here. (Rationales and full citations appear in the clinical practice recommendations and rationale section of this document.)

SKIN ASSESSMENT

Risk factor scales such as the Braden Q do not predict risk for device-related pressure ulcers. Because pressure ulcers from devices are the most common pressure-related injuries in the neonatal period, it is necessary to be aware of which devices are often involved (such as nasal continuous positive airway pressure [NCPAP] equipment), and to assess skin condition frequently.

BATHING

Several studies have shown the benefits of immersion bathing for the newborn's first bath, even with the umbilical cord in place, including for the late preterm infant. Water and mild liquid baby wash have similar effects on selected skin parameters during the first month of life.

DIAPER DERMATITIS

An assessment tool to help nurses evaluate diaper dermatitis and determine skin care treatment is included in Appendix B.

DISINFECTANTS

The U.S. Food and Drug Administration (FDA) has issued a labeling change to manufacturers of skin antiseptics containing chlorhexidine gluconate (CHG). The new label warns that CHG-containing skin antiseptics should be used with caution in premature infants or infants less than 2 months of age, as these products may cause chemical burns. At the same time, case reports of CHG/alcohol skin disinfectants and dressings causing skin injuries are becoming more frequent; therefore, the selection of skin disinfectants for extremely premature infants remains a dilemma for clinicians.

MEDICAL ADHESIVES

New technologies to decrease skin injury from medical adhesives include silicone adhesives and dressings and alcohol-free skin protectants. Silicone-based adhesive removers have been introduced that appear promising; however, further study is needed to determine both their safety and efficacy in neonates.

PRODUCT SELECTION CONSIDERATIONS

An appendix is included in this edition to offer clinicians general information that can facilitate decision-making or patient discussions about selection of topical skin care products for neonates (see Appendix C).

Conclusion

Protecting the newborn's delicate skin and promoting an intact and healthy skin barrier is challenging but important in the immediate neonatal period and may also contribute to skin health later in life. Understanding of the unique differences in neonatal and premature infant skin is necessary to provide daily care such as bathing, umbilical cord care, and applying emollients for dry skin. Even more challenging is protecting the skin integrity for hospitalized newborns exposed to skin disinfectants, medical adhesives, and devices such as NCPAP, monitors, and IV catheters.

The third edition of AWHONN's *Neonatal Skin Care Evidence-Based Clinical Practice Guideline* presents skin care recommendations based on current, published research in addition to seminal research studies. Future research about skin care practices—such as bathing and emollient use, the importance of the skin microbiome, and improvements in adhesive technology—is encouraged to expand the body of knowledge and support the commitment to evidence-based practice.

EVIDENCE-BASED CLINICAL PRACTICE GUIDELINE

Newborn Skin Assessment

	Clinical Practice	Referenced Rationale and Quality of Evidence Rating
1	Assess neonatal skin surfaces, head-to-toe, daily or more frequently as needed:	Routine assessment of skin is integral to providing good care and allows for assessment of risk for breakdown of skin integrity and for early identification and treatment of skin problems (**Lund, Kuller, et al., 2001: II-3**).
	• Recognize common transient benign skin conditions in the neonate.	Transient benign skin lesions include milia, erythema toxicum neonatorum, color changes from vascular instability, and desquamation. Knowledge of these benign lesions can help differentiate them from more serious cutaneous findings and provide reassurance to parents (**Lucky, 2008: III**).
2	Consider using a valid and reliable assessment tool to provide an objective measurement of skin condition, such as the following:	
	a. Skin Assessment: • Neonatal Skin Condition Score (NSCS)	The NSCS is an assessment tool that is used to evaluate skin condition in newborns, ranging from very-low-birthweight premature babies to full-term well babies (Appendix A). The NSCS's nine-point scale evaluates skin dryness, erythema, and breakdown (**Lund, Osborne, et al., 2001: II-3**). This tool was originally developed to evaluate overall skin condition in a sample of 2,820 infants in a large, multisite evidence-based practice project. Inter-rater reliability was evaluated in 16 sites with 475 assessments; intra-rater reliability was evaluated in 11 sites with 531 assessments. The NSCS is reliable when used by single and multiple raters to assess skin condition across weight and racial groups. Validity was confirmed by analyzing the relationship of the NSCS with birthweight, number of observations, and prevalence of infection. This scoring system can be integrated into skin care protocols to identify infants with excessive dryness, erythema that is potentially related to infections or irritations, and skin breakdown (**Lund & Osborne, 2004: II-2**).
	b. Risk Assessment: • Braden Q	The Braden Q and Starkid Skin Scale tools assess risk for pressure sores and skin breakdown in hospitalized pediatric patients. The Braden Q has been evaluated in two national surveys of pediatric pressure ulcer and skin breakdown prevalence. The scale evaluates seven categories: sensory perception, moisture, activity, mobility, nutrition, friction and shear, and tissue perfusion/oxygenation, with scores ranging from one to four for each (**Curley, Ramus, Roberts, & Wypij, 2003: II-2; McLane, Bookout, McCord, McCain, & Jefferson, 2004: II-2;**

Clinical Practice	Referenced Rationale and Quality of Evidence Rating
	Noonan, Quigley, & Curley, 2011: III; Suddaby, Barnett, & Facteau, 2005: II-2).
• Starkid Skin Scale	The Starkid Skin Scale, based on the Braden Q but simpler in format, was evaluated in 347 inpatient pediatric patients. The population studied included acute care as well as pediatric intensive care patients. Studies found that the majority of skin breakdown was caused by diaper dermatitis. The number of neonates in each study was not indicated, and patients of ages 0–12 months were included as a single group. No premature infants were included in these surveys (**Curley et al., 2003: II-2; McLane et al., 2004: II-2; Suddaby et al., 2005: II-2**). Immobility-related pressure ulcers in neonatal intensive care unit (NICU) patients are more likely to be identified in the early stage (erythema) and involve the occiput or ear. In studies of pediatric patients, pressure ulcers occurred more frequently in those receiving mechanical ventilation and among those with low mean arterial blood pressure (**Curley et al., 2003: II-2; McLane et al., 2004: II-2; Suddaby et al., 2005: II-2**). The authors of the Braden Q acknowledge that the Starkid Skin Scale tool can be used for neonates until a neonatal pressure ulcer risk assessment tool is developed and validated; they recommend using the Starkid Skin Scale for infants more than 3 weeks old and children up to 8 years old. They also note that the Braden Q does not predict device-related pressure sores, such as those seen with NCPAP, pulse oximeters, or IV hubs. Because these are the more commonly seen pressure ulcers in the NICU, vigilant observation and intervention for patients requiring these devices is necessary (**Noonan, et al., 2011: III**).
• Neonatal Skin Risk Assessment Scale (NSRAS)	The NSRAS was pilot-tested in 32 neonates and found to have limited reliability and validity, being most useful in predicting on which days in their observation period skin breakdown was most likely to occur. No further studies regarding the use of this tool in a larger population have been published (**Huffines & Logsdon, 1997: II-1**).
3 Identify risk factors for skin injury based on individual patient assessment. Risk factors may include but are not limited to the following: a. Gestational age less than 32 weeks b. Edema c. Dehydration d. Immobility due to illness, medications e. Use of vasopressors	The AWHONN/NANN RBP4 identified a series of items with potential for skin injury that were significantly related to higher skin scores using the NSCS tool (**Lund, Osborne, et al., 2001: II-3**). Premature infants are at risk for skin injury as a result of underdevelopment of the stratum corneum, diminished cohesion between epidermis and dermis, decreased collagen in the dermis, and edema (**Holbrook, 1982: III**). The two main causes of pressure ulcers in the neonatal population are immobility and medical devices. Examples of immobility-related pressure ulcers include newborns on assisted ventilation (**McLane et al., 2004: II-2**) and newborns on ECMO (**Harris, Coker, Smith, Uitvlugt, & Doctor, 2003: III**).

	Clinical Practice	Referenced Rationale and Quality of Evidence Rating
	f. Use of endotracheal tubes, nasogastric or orogastric tubes, vascular access devices, monitors, electrodes, probes g. Surgical wound h. Ostomies i. Nasal CPAP j. High-frequency ventilators k. Extracorporeal membrane oxygenation (ECMO) l. Prolonged electroencephalographic (EEG) monitoring	Routine rotation of devices such as blood pressure cuffs, pulse oximetry probes, temperature probes, and continuous EEG recording mechanisms is necessary to prevent pressure ulcers (**Baharestani, 2007: III**).
4	Determine potential causes of skin breakdown and skin injury, such as the following: a. Adhesive removal b. Burn/thermal injury c. Abrasion/friction d. Diaper dermatitis e. Pressure ulcer f. Infection g. Cooling blanket	Determining the potential cause of skin breakdown may help in decision-making about the optimal treatment regimen and may lead to strategies to prevent further skin disruption (**Lund, Kuller, Lane, Lott, & Raines, 1999: III**). Although no direct link between whole body cooling for hypoxic-ischemic encephalopathy and subcutaneous fat necrosis (SCFN), clinicians are reporting cases in greater numbers in the neonatal population. Nodules appear days to weeks after the initial insult and are described as erythematous, mobile nodules on the back, trunk, buttocks, arms, thighs, and cheeks. The exact pathophysiology of SCFN remains unknown, and it is also not known whether it is preventable. Potential complications of SCFN may include hypercalcemia, thrombocytopenia, hypoglycemia, hypertriglyceridemia, inflammatory cascade, and subcutaneous atrophy; the lesions may also be painful. Subcutaneous fat necrosis generally resolves in weeks to months (**Woods & Cederholm, 2012: III**). For further details, refer to the "Skin Breakdown" section of this Guideline.

Bathing

	Clinical Practice	Referenced Rationale and Quality of Evidence Rating
	General Newborn Bathing Principles	
1	Implement a hand hygiene policy for staff and visitors that includes hand cleansing with a facility-approved antibacterial cleanser before bathing infants. • Use a standardized hand-washing procedure such as the Centers for Disease Control and Prevention (CDC) guidance for hand hygiene in health care settings.	Transmission of community-acquired infections, including MRSA, can be prevented with adherence to standard infection control measures, including hand hygiene and environmental cleaning (CDC, 2006: III; Watson, 2006: II-3). Hand hygiene before and after patient contact is the most important practice in the prevention of hospital-acquired infections (**American Academy of Pediatrics [AAP] & American College of Obstetricians and Gynecologists [ACOG], 2012: III; CDC, 2013: III**).
2	Use standard precautions, including wearing gloves, until after the newborn's first bath.	Maternal blood and blood-stained amniotic fluid may pose a threat to health care professionals. Neonates should be considered contaminated with blood-borne pathogens until they are cleansed of blood and amniotic fluid (**Blume-Peytavi et al., 2009: III; CDC, 2006: III; Da Cunha, Procianoy, Franceschini, De Oliveira, & Cunha, 2008: I**). Removal of blood and secretions from the newborn may help to minimize the risk of infection (**AAP & ACOG, 2012: III**).
3	Ensure that bath equipment is disinfected before and after each use.	Bathing equipment can harbor microorganisms. Cleaning and disinfecting the tub is necessary for decontamination (**AAP & ACOG, 2012: III**).
4	Implement environmental controls to create a neutral thermal environment and to minimize neonatal heat loss during bathing, including the following: a. Ensure that bath water temperature ranges from 38°C to less than 40°C (100°F to <104°F). b. Consider using a thermometer to assess water temperature before bathing. c. Ensure that the room temperature is 26–27°C (79–81°F).	Bathing is a significant factor influencing thermoregulation during the early neonatal period, especially for infants born prior to 37 completed weeks of gestation (**Loring et al., 2012: I**). With appropriate environmental controls, heat loss during bathing is minimized, regardless of setting, timing, or provider (**Medves & O'Brien, 2004: I; Nako et al., 2000: I**).

	Clinical Practice	Referenced Rationale and Quality of Evidence Rating
	d. Close the door in the room where bathing takes place to minimize air currents and convective heat loss. e. Use prewarmed towels for drying.	
5	Use warm tap water for bathing.	Water has limits in cleansing efficacy (**Adam, Schnetz, Mathey, Pericoi, & De Prost, 2009: II-1**). The use of water versus soap-and-water baths demonstrated no difference in the bacterial colonization of the skin after the bath in both premature and full-term newborns (**Da Cunha & Procianoy, 2005: I**). Bathing with mild cleanser compared with bathing with water alone has minimal effect on skin bacterial colonization. Skin colonization increases over time, regardless of use of cleansers (**Medves & O'Brien, 2001: I**). No difference in the Transepidermal water loss (TEWL) measurement was found between babies bathed in water alone vs. with a cleansing product. The researchers concluded that the baby wash used in this study, or other technically equivalent cleansers, would not disrupt skin barrier integrity (**Lavender et al., 2013: I**).
	General Considerations for Preterm Infants	
1	For preterm infants less than 32 weeks of gestation, gently clean skin surfaces using warm water only during the first week of life. Use soft materials such as cotton cloth or cotton balls. Avoid rubbing; water can be squeezed onto the skin during rinsing. If areas of skin breakdown are evident, use warm sterile water.	Preterm infants have an immature stratum corneum and overall underdeveloped skin structures and are at risk for skin disruption and toxicity from topically applied substances (**Mancini, 2004: III**). The bathing schedule for preterm infants should be based on the infant's physiological condition and behavioral state (**Liaw, Yang, Yuh, & Yin, 2006: II-3; Peters, 1998: II-1**).
2	Preterm infants should usually not be bathed daily.	

	Clinical Practice	Referenced Rationale and Quality of Evidence Rating
	General Considerations for Choosing Cleansers	
1	Use skin cleansers with the least irritating formulation.	Cleansers emulsify oil, dirt, and microorganisms on the skin surface so they can be more easily removed. Only about 65% of oil and dirt on the skin can be removed with water alone. (**Kuehl, Fyfe, & Shear, 2003: III**). A mild baby wash is more effective than water at removing components of feces and urine from the skin surface (**Blume-Peytavi et al., 2009: III**). A randomized, controlled trial of 180 healthy infants showed improved skin hygiene and reduced skin irritation when a mild cleanser was used rather that water alone for bathing (**Dizon, Galzote, Estanislao, Mathew, & Sarkar, 2010: I**).
	a. Select mild cleansing bars or liquid cleansers that have a neutral or mildly acidic pH (5.5–7.0) or those that have minimal impact on the baby's skin surface pH.	Soap-based cleansers generally have a higher likelihood of drying or irritating skin and compromising the skin barrier, particularly when used under hard-water conditions. Water hardness, determined by the dissolved mineral content, can affect how skin reacts to different cleansing products. The pH of the skin surface and the degree of water hardness have been linked to atopic dermatitis in children (**Blume-Peytavi et al., 2009: III; Ertel, 2003: III; Hopkins, 2004: III; Kuehl et al., 2003: III**). A higher pH of the skin surface has also been related to increased bacterial proliferation on the skin (Garcia Bartels et al., 2010: I).
	b. Ideally, a cleanser should not: • cause skin irritation,	Soap made with lye is alkaline (pH >7.0), whereas mild cleansing bars, including synthetic detergent bars, and mild liquid cleansers are formulated to a mildly acidic pH (5.5–7.0) (**Gfatter et al., 1997: I**). Liquid cleansers generally cause less skin irritation and less disruption of the skin barrier, normal pH, and acid mantle, and they rinse more easily than soap (**Gfatter et al., 1997: I; Kuehl et al., 2003: III; Sarkar, Basu, Agrawal, & Gupta, 2010: III**).
	• disrupt the normal pH of the skin, or	The irritation potential of soaps may be attributed to their alkalinity (**Dizon et al., 2010: I; Tyebkhan, 2002: III**) and is also a direct reflection of the presence of surfactants in soaps (**Korting & Braun-Falco, 1996: III**). Solutions with a high pH can increase stratum corneum swelling and the potential for skin damage (**Ananthapadmanabhan, Moore, Subramanyan, Misra, & Meyer, 2004: III**).
	• cause stinging or irritation of the eyes.	An infant's blink reflex is present at birth but is much slower than in adults. Defensive blinking is essential to protect the eyes from injury and is not a fully reliable response until about 4 months of age (**Kayed, Farstad, & van der Meer, 2008: II-1**).
2	Choose products containing preservatives that have demonstrated safety and tolerability in newborns.	Preservatives are usually necessary in liquid soaps or cosmetics with high water content to prevent the overgrowth of microorganisms that may occur with regular use. However, these may be the cause of allergic irritant or contact dermatitis (**Blume-Peytavi et al., 2009: III; Lundov, Moesby, Zachariae, & Johansen, 2009: III; Tyebkhan, 2002: III**).

Bathing

	Clinical Practice	Referenced Rationale and Quality of Evidence Rating
3	Avoid antimicrobial soaps whenever possible.	Antimicrobial soap is not recommended for use in neonates because of the harshness of the soap as well as the potentially negative effect it may have on normal skin colonization. The effects of a product on the newborn skin should be considered in product selection of hospitalized newborns (**AAP & ACOG, 2012: III**).
	Bathing Procedure	
1	Bathe the infant according to facility protocols. The following methods of bathing are used:	
	a. Sponge-bathing: Place the infant on a soft surface. • Keep the infant wrapped in a towel. • Gently expose one body part at a time for cleansing and rinsing.	Sponge-bathing—washing with a cloth from a small basin of warm water—may cause increased heat loss leading to cold stress, which can contribute to crying and agitation of the newborn (**Cole, Brissette, & Lunardi, 1999: III**). Physiologic (heart rate and oxygen saturation) and behavioral disruptions (distress cues) have been reported during sponge-bathing of preterm infants; therefore, routine sponge-bathing is not recommended for ill premature infants (**Peters, 1998: II-I**).
	b. Tub (immersion)-bathing: • Fill the tub with water deep enough to keep the infant's shoulders covered. • Hold the infant firmly under the buttocks and the back of the neck and gently lower her or his body, except head and neck, into the water. • Wash the infant's face first with warm water and a clean cloth. • Wash the rest of the body from the top down. • Gently rinse the infant.	Gently placing the infant feet-first into the tub and covering the entire body with water ensures an even temperature distribution and decreases evaporative heat loss (**Anderson, Lane, & Chang, 1995: II-I**). When compared with sponge-bathing, infants bathed in a tub showed a reduction in crying and inducement of a calm, quiet state. In addition, maternal pleasure and confidence were greater with immersion bathing of their infants when compared with sponge-bathing (**Bryanton, Walsh, Barrett, & Gaudet, 2004: I; Cole et al., 1999: III**). No differences in bacterial colonization of the cord, cord infection, or frequency of diaper dermatitis were found among infants who were immersed in water compared with sponge-bathed infants (**Henningson, Nystrom & Tunnel, 1981: I; Bryanton et al., 2004: I; Garcia Bartels et al, 2009: I; Loring et al., 2012: I**). Because routine tub-bathing has been shown to cause stress symptoms in hospitalized preterm infants, whenever possible, tub bath routines should be modified to match the infant's developmental patterns and growth (**Liaw, et al., 2006: II-3**).

	Clinical Practice	Referenced Rationale and Quality of Evidence Rating
	c. Swaddled bathing: • Place the infant in a flexed, midline position, swaddled in a blanket or soft towel. • Immerse the infant in a tub of warm water. • Unwrap and gently wash one body part at a time.	Infants may experience uncontrolled motor activity when placed in a bathtub. Swaddled bathing promotes a secure feeling. Swaddled bathing allows the infant to remain in a contained position during the entire bath and decreases random movements. Parental stress may also be reduced because swaddled bathing promotes a quiet-calm newborn state (**Fern, Graves, & L'Huillier, 2002: III**).
2	After bathing:	
	a. Dry the infant, immediately diaper, place cap on her or his head, and wrap in warm blankets.	Infants frequently cry when they are removed from the warm bath, and their skin temperature cools rapidly. Having warm towels ready will help prevent cooling and decrease crying. Newborn skin is sensitive and susceptible to trauma (**Sarkar et al., 2010: III**).
	b. Within approximately 10 minutes after the first bath, dress the infant, change the cap, and wrap her or him in dry, warm blankets.	Significant neonatal temperature decreases have been reported to occur 10 minutes after the first bath. Clothing placed on the infant immediately after the bath can become damp and a source of rapid evaporative heat loss (**Anderson et al., 1995: II-1; Medves & O'Brien, 2004: I; Varda & Behnke, 2000: I**).
	c. If skin dryness, flaking, or cracking are apparent after bathing, an emollient may be applied.	Emollients have been shown to protect the integrity of the skin barrier (**Blume-Peytavi et al., 2009: III**).
	First Bath	
1	Give the first bath once the neonate has achieved thermal and cardiorespiratory stability. It is ideal to wait at least 2 hours, whenever possible.	At birth, the skin of newborns enters a process of adaptation. Many controversies exist about skin care in newborns, particularly whether healthy, full-term babies should be bathed or washed during the first week of life. Regimens vary in frequency, use of water or cleansing agents, bathing procedures (tub or sponge), and the appropriate age in hours for giving the first bath (**Garcia Bartels et al., 2009: I**). Bathing full-term infants immediately following birth can potentially compromise thermal and cardiorespiratory stability during transition. When environmental controls are implemented, bathing does not compromise neonatal thermal stability (**Blume-Peytavi, et al., 2009: III; Bryanton et al., 2004: I; Nako et al., 2000: I**).

Bathing

	Clinical Practice	Referenced Rationale and Quality of Evidence Rating
2	For full-term infants who are not compromised, bathe after axillary temperature is 36.8°C or more (≥98.2°F) and the infant is at least 1 hour of age.	Bathing the full-term newborn with an axillary temperature of 36.8°C or more (≥98.2°F) after 1 hour of age has not been shown to compromise neonatal thermal stability and may reduce health care providers' exposure to blood-borne pathogens (**Behring, Vezeau, & Fink, 2003: I; Varda & Behnke, 2000: I**).
3	For the late preterm infant (34 0/7–36 6/7 weeks of gestation), postponing the first bath until thermal stability is reached (approximately 2–4 hours after birth) is recommended.	Late preterm infants have thinner skin and a larger ratio of surface area to weight, less insulating white adipose tissue, and less heat-generating brown fat. They have an increased risk of mortality and morbidity, especially complications associated with cold stress, when compared with term infants (**AWHONN, 2010: III; Engle, Tomashek, Wallman, & AAP Committee on Fetus and Newborn, 2007: III; Loring, et al., 2012: I**).
4	Bathing may be performed at the bedside or in the nursery when the environmental controls outlined above are implemented.	With appropriate environmental controls, there is no difference in heat loss whether the first bath is at the bedside by the parent or in the nursery by the nurse (**Medves & O'Brien, 2004: I**). Bathing can provide tactile stimulation for the newborn and a bonding opportunity for parents and caregivers (**Bryanton et al., 2004: I**).
5	Keep the duration of the bath as short as possible. • 5–10 minutes is typically an adequate length of time for the bath.	Sponge-bathing changes the infant's physiologic parameters, including temperature. Therefore, short baths based on assessment of the individual infant's physiologic stability are recommended (**Tapia-Rombo, Morales-Mora, & Alvarez-Vazquez, 2003: III**). Some clinicians prefer limiting the bath to 5 minutes to prevent cold stress and limit exposure to soap (**Blume-Peytavi et al., 2009: III**).
6	Use warm tap water and a minimal amount of pH-neutral or slightly acidic cleanser to assist with removal of blood and amniotic fluid. a. Use of tap water is safe unless there are known concerns about the quality of the water supply.	 No specific scientific evidence identifies the preferred source of water for neonatal bathing. However, a number of researchers have used tap water in studying bathing practices for both term and preterm neonates (**Bryanton et al., 2004: I; Da Cunha & Procianoy, 2005: I; Nako et al., 2000: I**).

Clinical Practice	Referenced Rationale and Quality of Evidence Rating
b. Infants with significant breaks in skin integrity may benefit from being bathed in warmed sterile water. If sterile water is used, appropriate methods to warm the water and confirm the correct temperature is achieved before bathing are necessary.	Sterile water reduces risk of contamination with microorganisms when skin integrity is altered (**Lund & Kuller, 2007: III**).
7 Leave vernix on the skin. If contaminated with blood, meconium, or other intrauterine debris, gently remove the contaminate but do not vigorously scrub to remove all vernix.	Leaving vernix on the skin allows for earlier newborn skin acidification and the World Health Organization (WHO) guidelines for newborn care specify that vernix on the newborn's skin should not be removed (**Stokowski, 2006: III; WHO, 2006: III**). Additionally, vernix is an active and naturally occurring skin cleanser (**Moraille, Pickens, Visscher, & Hoath, 2005: II-1**). The use of soap and vigorous scrubbing to remove vernix can result in skin damage. The protein components of vernix have protective properties against certain bacterial and fungal organisms that are lost if the vernix is removed (**Medves & O'Brien, 2001: I**). Refer also to the "Vernix" section of this Guideline.
Routine Bathing Bathe the infant every few days using appropriate safety measures. *1* Bathe to remove debris and for general hygiene purposes.	
a. Bathing is not an innocuous procedure. The benefits of daily bathing have not been clearly justified.	Bathing introduces acute and unexpected changes in stratum corneum with water interaction, potentially leading to drier skin surface (**Visscher et al., 2002: II-1**).
b. Under normal circumstances, neonates need not be bathed more frequently than approximately every other day.	Less frequent bathing minimizes behavioral and physiologic instability of premature infants, as a result of less handling and cold stress. In a randomized, controlled study of preterm infants, bathing every fourth day did not result in a significant increase in the number of skin flora or colony counts when compared with bathing every other day. No infants in either group developed an infection as a result of the frequency of bathing (**Quinn, Newton, & Piecuch, 2005: I**).

Clinical Practice	Referenced Rationale and Quality of Evidence Rating
• Decisions about the frequency of bathing and time of day should be based on the individual neonate's needs and consideration of family beliefs and values of the local culture.	Individualized assessment of infants and their families is needed so that bathing practices better address their concerns (**Tapia-Rombo et al., 2003: III**). Evening bathing may help to calm the baby and improve sleep (**Blume-Peytavi et al., 2009: III**).
c. Shampooing once or twice a week is usually adequate. Massage the entire scalp gently, including the area over the fontanelles.	Shampoos should meet the same safety requirements as those of a baby wash and should demonstrate eye mildness (**Blume-Peytavi et al., 2009: III**).
2 Educate parents and family members about bathing safety, including but not limited to the following guidance:	
a. Place the bathtub in a safe place on a sturdy surface. Never leave the baby alone or with other children during bathing.	The baby should never be left alone while in the bath, even if a bath seat is used. Young children should not be allowed to wash the baby (**Blume-Peytavi et al., 2009: III**).
b. Lower the water temperature of the water heater. Mix bath water to ensure an even temperature and check water before placing the baby into it.	Full thickness scald burns can occur to adults within 5 seconds at 140° and to children with even briefer exposure. Parents should be educated to lower their water heater temperature to below 120° (**Spencer, Shileds, & Smith, 2005: III**).
c. Selection of baby bathing products	Select bathing products that are mild and nonirritating to the skin and eyes (**Blume-Peytavi et al., 2009: III**).

Clinical Practice	Referenced Rationale and Quality of Evidence Rating
Special Needs in Developing Countries	
• Consider the topical use of CHG cleanser for newborn bathing and skin care in developing countries.	Morbidity and mortality continues to be a concern for newborns in developing countries. Chlorhexidine is often used because of its effectiveness against gram-positive and gram-negative bacteria. One study of 93 full-term infants found reduced S. aureus colonization 24 hours after the CHG bath when compared with infants bathed with a mild, neutral cleanser (**Da Cunha et al., 2008: I**). The use of 0.25% CHG wipes, normal saline washing, or no skin care was evaluated in 60 preterm (28–36 weeks), low-birthweight infants (1,001–2,000 g). Axillary colonization was reduced at 24 hours for those infants washed with CHG wipes; however, there was no difference in axillary colonization at 72 hours of age (**Sankar et al., 2009: I**). One study of 286 newborns in Nepal compared skin culture rates on newborns that were cleansed with various concentrations of CHG solutions. At 2 hours of age, all newborns had a reduction in positive skin cultures; however, the overall skin cultures at 24 hours of age were only lower when higher concentrations of CHG were used (**Mullany et al., 2008: I**). Another study of 133 newborns in Bangladesh compared skin cultures with CHG cleansing versus placebo cleansing. Positive skin culture results in the axillary, periumbilical, and inguinal areas were lower at various timed measurements in those infants in the CHG cleansing group (**Darmstad, Hossain, et al., 2007: I**). One small study of 12 children (ages 3 months to 12 years) showed small concentrations of CHG in the blood but no evidence that repeated exposure led to CHG accumulation in the blood (**Lee et al., 2011: II-1**).

	Clinical Practice	Referenced Rationale and Quality of Evidence Rating
1	Residual vernix does not need to be removed after birth. It can be left in place and allowed to wear off with normal care and handling.	Vernix is a fetal protective skin film, unique to humans, that acts as a chemical and mechanical barrier in utero and facilitates postnatal adaptation to an extrauterine dry environment. Vernix production begins at the end of the second trimester and accumulates on fetal skin in a cephalocaudal manner (**Haubrich, 2003: III**). Vernix detaches from the skin as the levels of pulmonary surfactant rise, resulting in a progressive increase in the turbidity of the amniotic fluid (**Hoath & Pickens, 2003: III; Moraille et al., 2005: II-2; Narendran, Wickett, Pickens, & Hoath, 2000: II-2**). Vernix is composed of 80% water, 10% lipids and 10% proteins (**Rissmann et al., 2008: II-1; Tollin et al., 2005: II-1**). Surface distribution depends on gestational age, type of birth, birthweight, race, gender, and the presence of meconium (**Visscher et al., 2005: I**). After birth, vernix is thought to affect skin hydration and therefore should be allowed to dry naturally over time (**Rissmann et al., 2008: II-1**). The goal of the first bath should be to remove unwanted soil such as blood and meconium and to leave residual vernix intact. The WHO recommends leaving residual vernix intact after initial drying in the delivery room (**WHO, 2006: III**). In clinical care, vernix has been thought of as an unwanted soil, but recent research has shown vernix may play multiple roles (**Moraille et al., 2005: II-2**).
2	Be aware of and provide education to parents, where appropriate, about the functions and potential benefits of vernix for the newborn:	
	a. Protection against infection	The epidermal barrier is the first line of protection against bacterial cutaneous infection. Vernix contains antimicrobial peptides and proteins that are active against common bacterial and fungal pathogens and therefore have a direct role in defense against bacteria (**Larson & Dinulos, 2005: III; Tollin et al., 2005: II-1**). Recent studies identified a collection of surfactant proteins in vernix that are known to be important for airway sterility. They also suggest that these proteins fulfill a vital antimicrobial role in protection against intrauterine infection and postnatally until bacterial colonization of the gut occurs (**Akinbi, Narendran, Pass, Markart, & Hoath, 2004: II-3; Haubrich, 2003: III**).
	b. Decreased skin permeability and TEWL	Prenatally, vernix "waterproofs" the fetus and allows for epidermal growth free from the potential maceration caused by extended amniotic fluid exposure (**Yoshio, Lagercrantz, Gudmundsson, & Agerbeth, 2004: II-1; Youssef, Wickett, & Hoath, 2001: II-1**). In preterm infants, the stratum corneum functions poorly, which leads to high levels of TEWL. Application of topical ointments containing petrolatum improves preterm infants' barrier function and skin condition (**Nopper et al., 1996: I**). In one adult study, vernix was applied as a topical barrier cream and compared with

Clinical Practice	Referenced Rationale and Quality of Evidence Rating
	commercial topical emollients and petrolatum. Vernix treatment resulted in immediate increases in baseline surface hydration, moisture accumulation, and water-holding capacity greater than the other ointments (**Bautista, Wickett, Visscher, Pickens, & Hoath, 2000: II-1**). Application of synthetic vernix has been studied and may be an effective therapy to enhance epidermal barrier formation and function (**Tansirikongkol, Visscher, & Wickett, 2007: II-I**).
c. Skin cleansing	In a study to test various cleansers' ability to remove test soil from adult forearms, vernix exhibited a cleansing capability comparable or superior to standard skin cleansers (**Hoath & Pickens, 2003: III; Moraille et al., 2005: II-2**).
d. Moisturization of the skin surface	Vernix contains 80% water, while petrolatum jelly contains 0.03% water. For this reason, vernix has been called a naturally occurring barrier cream with moisturizing capacity. It functions as a moisturizer by increasing skin hydration and water-holding capacity, which helps to maintain the suppleness and plasticity of the stratum corneum (**Haubrich, 2003: III; Hoath, Narendran, & Visscher, 2001: III; Tansirikongkol et al., 2007: III; Visscher et al., 2011: II-1; Youssef et al., 2001: II-1**).
e. pH development	After birth, the skin surface pH drops from a neutral pH to an acidic pH, forming the acid mantle. The acid mantle inhibits the growth of pathogenic bacteria (**Larson & Dinulos, 2005: III**). The presence of vernix produces earlier acidification of the skin and may facilitate colonization by the normal flora after birth (**Tollin et al., 2005: II-1; Visscher et al., 2005: I**).
f. Wound healing	Vernix is important for epidermal barrier formation and rejuvenation after wounding of the skin (**Haubrich, 2003: III**). Glutamine, which constitutes greater than 20% of the amino acids in vernix, is a known trophic factor for the gut and is required by rapidly proliferating cells (**Hoath et al., 2001: III**). Early studies raise the possibility of using vernix as the prototype of a new barrier cream to facilitate the formation of an effective stratum corneum (**Tansirikongkol et al., 2007: II-1; Visscher et al., 2005: I**).
g. Temperature regulation	In one study, leaving vernix intact had no effect on axillary temperatures during the first hour after birth in older preterm infants (greater than 32 weeks of gestation) (**Visscher et al., 2005: I**).

Clinical Practice	Referenced Rationale and Quality of Evidence Rating
Immediate	
1 Clean the umbilical cord and surrounding skin surface as part of the initial bath. a. Wash the umbilical area with tap water to remove debris. b. Use cleanser sparingly if needed to remove debris. c. Dry thoroughly to remove excess moisture. d. Leave umbilical area and clamped umbilical cord stump clean, dry, and uncovered.	The umbilical cord of the newborn is a potential portal of entry for invasive bacterial pathogens (**Dinulos & Pace, 2008: III**). The routine use of antimicrobial sprays, creams, or powders for cord care has not been shown to be more effective in preventing infection than keeping the infant's cord clean and dry at birth (**AAP & ACOG, 2012: III; Zupan, Garner, & Omari, 2004: I**). Bathing does not delay cord healing or increase infection rate (**Bryanton et al., 2004: I**).
2 Implement standard precautions, including wearing gloves before touching or caring for the umbilical cord stump and surrounding area and before cleansing the infant. After the initial cleansing, implement standard infection control measures, including hand hygiene.	Transmission of community-acquired infections, including MRSA, can be prevented with adherence to standard infection-control measures, including hand hygiene (**CDC, 2006: III; Watson, 2006: II-3**).
Ongoing	
1 Use natural drying for umbilical cord care. Natural drying involves keeping the cord area clean and dry, without the routine application of topical agents.	Cord separation time is shorter for full-term neonates receiving natural drying (dry cord care) when compared with those receiving isopropyl alcohol to the cord on a daily basis (8.1 vs. 9.8 days) (**Dore et al., 1998: I**). Application of topical drying agents or antibiotics has demonstrated no beneficial effect on cord separation time or frequency of cord infections (**Medves & O'Brien, 1997: I; Zupan et al., 2004: I**).
2 The following steps should be implemented when providing cord care: a. Keep umbilical cord area clean and dry.	In preterm infants, cord separation time was reported to be shorter with natural drying (13 days) compared with alcohol care (16 days). Natural drying prevents exposure to isopropyl alcohol and the potential skin breakdown from chemical irritation (**Evens, George, Angst, & Schweig, 2004: I**). One study reported that infants receiving dry cord care (natural drying) may have more exudate and odor as compared with infants treated with

Clinical Practice	Referenced Rationale and Quality of Evidence Rating
b. Maintain aseptic technique to minimize contamination by pathogens. c. Wash hands before handling umbilical stump. d. Keep umbilical stump exposed to air or loosely covered with clean clothes. e. Keep diaper folded down and away from umbilical stump to prevent contamination with urine or stool. f. If the umbilical cord stump becomes soiled with urine or stool, cleanse the area with water. g. After cleansing with water, dry thoroughly with clean absorbent gauze to remove excess moisture, and then discard the gauze.	triple dye and alcohol protocols and had a higher colonization rate with microorganisms but no increase in infections (**Janssen, Selwood, Dobson, Peacock, & Thiessen, 2003: I**).
3 Discourage the routine use of the following antimicrobial topical agents:	The use of antimicrobial topical agents is not supported in the literature (**Zupan et al., 2004: I**).
a. Isopropyl alcohol	Isopropyl alcohol prolongs cord separation time and does not decrease bacterial colonization or infection rates (**Dore et al., 1998: I**). In a high-humidity, subtropical country, cord separation time was significantly decreased with natural drying when compared with cleansing with 95% alcohol, and the incidence of cord infection was not increased (**Hsu et al., 2010: I**). A comparison of triple dye application at birth plus routine isopropyl alcohol with triple dye application alone showed no difference in time to cord separation (**Suliman et al., 2010: I**).
b. Topical antimicrobial/antibacterial agents, including but not limited to povidone-iodine, CHG, and triple antibiotic ointment	Because of the developmental immaturity of neonatal skin, the potential for absorption and toxicity from antimicrobial/antibacterial agents is increased. Topical antimicrobials have been associated with allergic contact dermatitis and, rarely, anaphylaxis (**Chamnanvanakij, Decharachakul, Rasamimaree, & Vanprapar, 2005: I; Donlon & Furdon, 2002: III; Guala et al., 2003: II-2; Pezzati et al., 2003: I**).
c. Triple dye (brilliant green, crystal violet, and proflavine hemisulfate).	Triple dye can cause skin necrosis if it is inadvertently applied to the skin surrounding the umbilical stump. Cords treated with triple dye had the longest separation time when compared with dry cord care and alcohol cord care (**Chamnanvanakij et al., 2005: I**). Infants who received initial cord care with triple dye followed by alcohol had a longer time to cord

Clinical Practice	Referenced Rationale and Quality of Evidence Rating
	separation than infants who received only alcohol applied to the cord (**Golombek, Brill, & Salice, 2002: II-2; Suliman et al., 2010: I**).
4 Differentiate normal umbilical cord healing from potential problems, including infectious and noninfectious conditions. Contact the primary care provider if signs of a potential problem are present.	Normal healing of the newborn umbilical cord may create a moist, gelatinous appearance. The isolated presentation of a moist, gelatinous-appearing cord has not been associated with infection. The stimulatory effect of bacteria on wound healing has long been recognized. All wounds are colonized, but not all wounds are infected. Bacteria are believed to help initiate the inflammatory or first stage of wound healing (**Donlon & Furdon, 2002: III; Mendenhall & Eichenfield, 2000: III**). Small amounts of cloudy mucoid material normally collect at the junction of the necrotic cord stump and abdominal skin and should not be misinterpreted as pus (**Brook, 2002: III**).
a. Examples of infectious conditions that may affect the umbilical cord include but are not limited to the following: • Omphalitis • Periumbilical erythema • Neonatal tetanus • Periumbilical necrotizing fasciitis	Infectious and noninfectious conditions of the cord may also be present and cause delayed cord separation. Conditions that place the newborn at risk of umbilical infections include a nonvaccinated mother, nonsterile delivery conditions, and unusual cord care practices (**Donlon & Furdon, 2002: III; Janssen et al., 2003: I**). Omphalitis is characterized by drainage from the umbilical stump or its base at the point of attachment to the abdominal wall. Secretions may be thin and serous, sanguineous or frankly purulent, and, at times, foul-smelling. Signs of inflammation of the tissues surrounding the cord support the diagnosis of omphalitis, which may also be associated with fever, lethargy, or poor feeding (**Brook, 2002: III**). Necrotizing fasciitis presents with a blue, gray, or black appearance of the skin and can rapidly progress to thrombosis (**Donlon & Furdon, 2002: III**).
b. Examples of noninfectious conditions that may affect the umbilical cord include but are not limited to the following: • Umbilical granuloma • Clear drainage and inflammation confined within the umbilical ring • Urachal anomalies	If separation of the umbilical cord is delayed beyond 2 weeks, systematic evaluation for infection, underlying immune disorders, or embryologic remnants that communicate with the bowel or bladder is indicated (**Donlon & Furdon, 2002: III**).

	Clinical Practice	Referenced Rationale and Quality of Evidence Rating
5	Educate staff and families about the normal mechanism of umbilical cord healing with the following principles: a. The umbilical cord should be kept clean as part of normal hygiene practices. b. Moist, gelatinous appearance may be normal. c. Redness, swelling, and drainage are abnormal findings. d. Do not pull on the cord stump; allow natural detachment to take place.	The umbilical cord typically appears moist and gelatinous and, at times, has a characteristic odor. The umbilical cord stump will change from yellowish green to brown to black as it dries out and eventually falls off. The mechanism of umbilical cord separation involves infarction, mechanical drying, collagenase activity, granulocyte influx, and aseptic necrosis (**Donlon & Furdon, 2002: III; Mendenhall & Eichenfield, 2000: III; Zupan et al., 2004: I**).
1	***Special Needs in Developing Countries*** Consider the topical use of CHG for cord care in developing countries. Chlorhexidine products may include solutions, gels, and powders.	In developing countries, umbilical cord infection is a major cause of neonatal morbidity and mortality. Mothers often deliver at home under unhygienic conditions and may live in areas in close proximity to animals and animal dung. The prevalence of neonatal tetanus, gram-negative sepsis, and omphalitis is higher. It is possible that different standards of practice are needed for developing countries, where standard hygiene practices are not currently met (**AAP & ACOG, 2012: III; Mullany, Darmstadt, & Tielsch, 2003: III**). The WHO recommendations for developing countries include using nothing on the cord stump, folding the diaper below the stump, and using soap-and-water solution to clean the cord if visibly soiled (**WHO, 2006: III**). However, these recommendations have been questioned by researchers conducting trials that compare various cord care regimens in countries lacking basic resources, including clean water (**Mullany et al., 2003: III; Mullany et al., 2006: I**). One study in Nepal showed a 75% reduction in omphalitis and a 24% reduction in mortality when using an initial bath with 0.25% CHG followed by single application of 4% CHG solution to the umbilical cord within the first 24 hours of life (**Mullany et al., 2006: I**). Another study in the same country compared CHG gel to aqueous CHG for cord stump care. The gel formulation resulted in a superior reduction in bacterial growth 24 hours after application of these products (**Hodgins et al., 2010: I**). A randomized, controlled trial of 9,741 newborns in Pakistan found the application of 4% CHG to the umbilical cord by trained birth assistants with continued daily application at home by family members resulted in a decreased risk of infection and a reduction in neonatal mortality when compared with infants having only dry cord care (**Soofi et al., 2012: I**).

	Clinical Practice	Referenced Rationale and Quality of Evidence Rating
		A study in Bangladesh showed a decrease in overall cord redness and pus when cleansing the cord with 4% CHG as soon as possible as a single application after home birth or when using the same solution as a daily application for 7 days after home birth when compared with dry cord care. The single-application group also demonstrated a decrease in overall neonatal mortality when compared with the other two groups (**Arifeen et al., 2012: I**).
2	Consider using breast milk as a substitute for other topical agents for umbilical cord care in developing countries.	Breast milk has been shown to be effective in reducing colonization compared with other topical agents and may be used effectively for umbilical cord care in developing countries (**Ahmadpour-Kacho, Zahedpasha, Hajian, Javadi, & Talebian, 2006: I; Vural & Sezer, 2006: II-2**).
3	Provide education on cord care strategies to health care professionals in developing countries.	A Sri Lankan study found that a comprehensive education program for health care professionals about evidence-based cord care can be an effective strategy in changing maternal behavior (**Senarath, Fernando, & Rodrigo, 2007: II-2**).

Circumcision Care

	Clinical Practice	Referenced Rationale and Quality of Evidence Rating
1	Take the following steps for site preparation and care before, during, and after the procedure: a. Prepare the site with skin disinfectant (see the "Disinfectants" section of this Guideline). b. Following the procedure, completely remove any disinfectant with sterile water or saline. c. Pay special attention to leg creases and the lower back and buttocks, where pools tend to form during the procedure.	For those who choose circumcision for their newborns, the benefits of circumcision include prevention of urinary tract infections, penile cancer, and transmission of some sexually transmitted infections, including HIV (**AAP & ACOG, 2012: III**). Despite concerns about community-acquired *S. aureus,* no relationship has been found between circumcision and MRSA infections in neonates (**Fortunov, Hulten, Hammerman, Mason, & Kaplan, 2006: II-3**).
2	When circumcision is performed, analgesia should be provided.	Sucrose given by mouth, swaddling, and acetaminophen administration may reduce the stress response but are not sufficient for operative pain when used alone. While anesthetic creams and local anesthesia provide some benefit, both dorsal penile blocks and ring blocks provide more effective analgesia (**AAP, 1999: III; AAP & ACOG, 2012: III**).
3	Following the procedure, cover the penis with petrolatum-impregnated gauze strips for 24 hours. • Lubricants and dressings should generally not be used if the procedure is performed with a plastic circumcision device, unless indicated.	Petrolatum promotes healing (**Ghadially, Halkier-Sorensen, & Elias, 1992: II-1**). Using single, prepackaged petrolatum-impregnated gauze strips may decrease the risk of bacterial contamination associated with multiple-use containers (**Brown-Trask, Van Sell, Carter, & Kindred, 2009: III; Gelbaum, 1993: III**). Dressings and petrolatum are usually not indicated when a plastic device has been used for circumcision, because they could cause the plastic shield to move out of place (**Brown-Trask et al., 2009: III; Kaufman, Clark, & Castro, 2001: III**).
4	The benefits of antimicrobial ointments should be evaluated relative to the potential for subsequent allergic contact dermatitis.	In studies of adults with minor surgical procedures, use of white petrolatum and bacitracin resulted in equally low infection rates; petrolatum ointment has a minimal risk for induction of local and systemic allergic reactions compared with topical antibiotic ointments (**Smack et al., 1996: I**). Bacitracin has been noted as one of the 12 most frequent allergens causing a positive patch test reaction in patients between the ages of 8 and 92 years (**Marks et al., 1995: II-2**).

Clinical Practice	Referenced Rationale and Quality of Evidence Rating
5 Educate staff and families about how to care for the newborn penis.	Soaps and cleansers can be irritating to healing tissue (**Darmstadt & Dinulos, 2000: III**). Petrolatum helps prevent the healing tissue from sticking to the diaper (**Brown-Trask et al., 2009: III**).
a. Circumcised penis • Cleanse with water only for the first 3–4 days to prevent irritation. • Apply petrolatum to any red or raw areas on the head or shaft of the penis with each diaper change.	
b. Uncircumcised penis • Foreskin should not be retracted or forced away from the tip of the penis during bathing or diaper care.	After birth, the foreskin is attached to the tip of the penis, but it will gradually separate over time. The foreskin does not usually retract completely for several years and therefore should not be forcibly retracted (**AAP & ACOG, 2012: III; Ressler-Maerlender & Sorensen, 2005: III**).

Disinfectants

	Clinical Practice	Referenced Rationale and Quality of Evidence Rating
1	Disinfect skin surfaces before invasive procedures, such as insertion of central venous catheters, placement of peripheral IV catheters, umbilical vessel catheterization, chest tube insertion, venipuncture, or heel sticks for laboratory samples.	Disinfecting skin surfaces with antiseptic solutions before invasive procedures reduces the risk of bacteremia, catheter-related infections, and skin contamination during blood culture sampling (**CDC, 2011: III; Polin, Denson, Brady, & AAP Committee on Fetus and Newborn and Committee on Infectious Diseases, 2012: III**). Colonization and infection of central catheters has been defined as *extraluminal* when the infection occurs shortly after the catheter is inserted or *intraluminal* when the catheter has been in place for a prolonged period of time. Infections arising from the extraluminal route can be prevented by effective cutaneous antisepsis at the insertion site. Infections from an intraluminal source can be prevented by strict adherence to aseptic technique for catheter hubs, caps, connectors, and IV tubing (**Mermel, 2011: III**).
2	Select a disinfectant by evaluating risks and benefits of each product relative to efficacy, potential for toxicity, and skin irritation. Evidence is insufficient to recommend a single product for all neonates.	
	a. Consider efficacy. • CHG	Chlorhexidine gluconate is a chlorinated cationic biguanide and is used in both aqueous solutions and in combination with isopropyl alcohol; its bactericidal properties increase cell membrane permeability, and it is effective against both gram-positive and gram-negative organisms. It also binds to protein in the stratum corneum of the epidermis, leaving a residual bactericidal effect that is resistant to alcohol removal (**Chapman, Aucott, & Milstone, 2012: III**). According to current FDA labeling regulations, some CHG/isopropyl alcohol-containing products are now labeled: "Use with care in premature infants or infants less than 2 months of age. These products may cause irritation or chemical burns" (**FDA, 2012: III**). However, NICUs may be using this product "off label" for infants less than 2 months of age as indicated for disinfection. In a survey of 100 NICU training programs, 61% of respondents used some form of CHG in infants under 2 months of age to reduce catheter-related blood infection (**Tamma, Aucott, & Milstone, 2010: III**). Despite the fact that a metaanalysis of eight studies involving a total of 4,143 catheters in adult patients determined that CHG-containing solutions used for insertion and catheter site care reduced the risk for catheter-related bloodstream infection by 49% (risk ratio, 0.51; confidence interval, 0.27–0.97) (**Chaiyakunapruk, Veenstra, Lipsky, & Saint, 2002: I**), current CDC guidelines indicate that there is insufficient evidence to make a recommendation about the safety or efficacy of CHG products in infants less than 2 months of age (**CDC, 2011: III**).

Clinical Practice	Referenced Rationale and Quality of Evidence Rating
• 2% aqueous CHG in 4-oz. bottles	In the United States, aqueous CHG products (2% and 4%) must be poured from bottles onto sterile gauze for application, although aqueous single-use products are available in other countries (**Andersen, Hart, Vemgal, & Harrison, 2005: II-2; Lashkari, Chow, & Godambe, 2012: III**). In adults, aqueous 2% CHG reduced catheter-related infections when compared with 10% povidone-iodine and 70% isopropyl alcohol (**Maki, Ringer, & Alvarado, 1991: I**).
• 0.5% CHG in 70% isopropyl alcohol	Use of 0.5% CHG in isopropyl alcohol reduces peripheral IV catheter colonization in premature and term newborns when compared with povidone-iodine (**Garland et al., 1995: II-3**). In a sequential study in a NICU, the rate of positive blood cultures, the number of true infections or contaminated cultures during the time when 10% povidone-iodine was used, was not statistically different from the second time when 0.5% CHG/70% isopropyl alcohol was used (**Linder et al., 2004: II-3**).
• 2% CHG in 70% isopropyl alcohol	A pilot trial of 47 infants weighing more than 1,500 grams and more than 7 days of age compared cutaneous tolerance of 2% CHG in 70% isopropyl alcohol to 10% povidone-iodine. There were no differences in number of blood stream infections or sepsis evaluations. This small study, however, was terminated by the sponsor because of slow enrollment and was not powered to look at the overall infection rates (**Garland et al., 2009: I**).
• 3.15% CHG in 70% isopropyl alcohol	Blood culture contaminants in a pediatric emergency department were significantly lower when skin was disinfected using 3.15% CHG in isopropyl alcohol compared with povidone-iodine (**Marlowe et al., 2010: II-2**).
• 10% povidone-iodine	Povidone-iodine is widely available in a 10% aqueous solution and in single-use wipes and applicators. It is more efficacious than isopropyl alcohol for skin disinfection (**Choudhuri, McQueen, Inoue, & Gordon, 1990: II-1; Maki et al., 1991: I**). In newborns, povidone-iodine has been shown to be less effective than CHG in reducing peripheral IV catheter colonization (**Garland et al., 1995: II-3**) and equally effective as CHG in reducing bacterial colony counts before IV catheter insertions (**Malathi, Miller, Leeming, Hedges, & Marlow, 1993: II-2**).
b. Consider potential for systemic toxicity if skin disinfectants are absorbed through the skin.	
• Povidone-iodine	If absorbed through the skin, povidone-iodine can cause alterations in thyroid function in premature and term newborns (**Khashu, Chessex, & Chanoine, 2005: III; Linder et al., 1997: II-3; Mitchell, Pollock, Jamieson, Fitzpatrick, & Logan, 1991: II-2; Parravicini et al., 1996: II-2; Smerdely et al., 1989: II-2**). However, two studies in the United States did not report alterations in thyroid function with povidone-iodine use. One study used povidone-iodine for skin disinfection in premature infants with a mean gestational age of 33 weeks; there was no evidence of abnormal thyroid

levels. However, it is important to note that the study's use of a single measurement of thyroid function, obtained on day 7–10 of life, may have been too soon to identify the systemic effects of iodine absorption (**Gordon, Rowitch, Mitchell, & Kohane, 1995: III**). Another study reported elevated urine iodine in 30 infants less than 30 weeks of gestation and transiently decreased T3 and T4 levels, while levels of thyroid-stimulating hormone did not rise. These findings may reflect a euthyroid state or normal thyroid physiology of prematurity (**AvRuskin, Greenfield, Prasad, Greig, Juan, 1994: II-1**). Another possible explanation for the difference between studies in the United States and those in other countries may be attributed to higher iodine intake during pregnancy in U.S. women.

- CHG-based preparations

Systemic CHG toxicity was not identified in the previously cited studies of CHG use in neonates in this Guideline. Chlorhexidine gluconate has been used for several decades in Europe and increasingly in the United States and Canada in the past 5 years in adults and children, including premature neonates. Chlorhexidine gluconate exposure has been implicated in rare cases of contact dermatitis and anaphylactic reactions in adults, particularly in CHG-impregnated devices, such as urinary catheters, or exposure to atopic skin (**Knight, Puy, Douglass, O'Hehir, & Thien, 2001: III**). A recent observational case series highlighted the association between the use of CHG-impregnated dressings and erosive contact dermatitis, even in young infants (**Weitz, 2013: III**).

A pilot trial to examine the cutaneous tolerance of 2% CHG in isopropyl alcohol in newborns under 32 weeks of gestation found measurable concentrations of CHG in 7 of the 10 infants who had levels drawn. However, there were no reported systemic effects. The role of isopropyl alcohol in combination with CHG may be a possible contributing factor to cutaneous absorption of CHG (**Garland et al., 2009: I**).

Chlorhexidine gluconate can be safely used on the scalp for IV or central line placement if applied judiciously, without splashing or excess solution, and should be completely removed after the procedure is complete (**Lund & Kuller, 2007: III**). There is no clinical data to discourage the use of CHG for skin preparation prior to lumbar puncture or epidural catheter placement (**Milstone, Passaretti, & Perl, 2008: III**).

c. Consider the potential for skin irritation, chemical burns, or erosive contact dermatitis.

Wound cleanser studies in human tissue cultures suggest that a number of cleansers, disinfectants, and liquid bath soaps can damage or destroy fibroblasts and keratinocytes in healing wounds; these findings may also be applicable to potential damage to neonatal skin, particularly for the premature neonate (**Wilson, Mills, Prather, & Dimitrijevich, 2005: II-1**).

A number of case reports document chemical burns from disinfectants containing 0.5% CHG in methanol (**Bringué Espuny et al., 2010: III; Reynolds, Banerjee, & Meek, 2005: III**), 0.5% CHG in 70% isopropyl alcohol (**Mannan, Chow, Lissauer, & Godambe, 2007: III**), and 2%

aqueous CHG (Andersen et al., 2005: II-2). Case reports indicating chemical burns from isopropyl alcohol and povidone-iodine solutions in extremely-low-birthweight infants are also reported (**Sardesai, Kornacka, Walas, & Ramanathan, 2011: III**).

A prospective study of 40 infants with a mean gestational age of 32 weeks (range: 23–39 weeks) found the use of 2% CHG in isopropyl alcohol for peripherally inserted central catheter insertion and weekly dressing changes compromised skin barrier function. This compromise was measured by elevated TEWL, erythema, and dryness (**Visscher, deCastro, et al., 2009: II-1**).

A pilot trial comparing 2% CHG in isopropyl alcohol in 47 premature infants weighing more than 1,500 grams and more than 7 days old found no increase in skin redness or breakdown when used for insertion and weekly dressing changes and only one incidence of erythema in a newborn treated with povidone-iodine disinfection (**Garland et al., 2009: I**).

Chlorhexidine gluconate has been associated with local reactions to a CHG patch dressing for central venous catheters in very-low-birthweight infants in a large, randomized, controlled trial involving 705 neonates; although the use of this dressing reduced catheter tip colonization, it did not change the rate of catheter-related blood stream infection and blood stream infection in this population (**Garland et al., 2001: I**). Case reports describe erosive irritant contact dermatitis resulting from CHG-impregnated transparent dressings applied to femoral catheters in children (**Weitz, 2013: III**).

---

3 Consider the following suggested techniques for applying disinfectants:

Guidelines from the CDC state that antiseptics should be allowed to dry according to the manufacturer's recommendation prior to inserting a central venous catheter (**CDC, 2011: III**). At present, no single product is recommended for all neonates.

a. Apply CHG for 30 seconds or with two consecutive applications. Aqueous CHG may not dry but can be wiped with sterile gauze after the application.

A small study of 11 infants with 25 peripheral catheters compared techniques of application of 0.5% CHG/isopropyl alcohol with povidone-iodine, using single- or double-swabbing and different time intervals ranging from 5 to 30 seconds. Two consecutive cleansings or a longer duration of cleansing is recommended for more effective skin sterilization (**Malathi et al., 1993: II-2**).

Chlorhexidine gluconate has been shown to be efficacious in reducing skin colonization at IV catheters in neonates (**Garland et al., 1995: II-3**) and catheter-related blood stream infections in adults (**Chaiyakunapruk et al., 2002: I; Maki et al., 1991: I**). However, CHG products with a single-use applicator that are currently available in the United States contain isopropyl alcohol and may result in chemical burns or skin irritation in premature infants.

	Clinical Practice	Referenced Rationale and Quality of Evidence Rating
		Aqueous 2% and 0.5% CHG products are available in other countries. However, even aqueous CHG products can potentially cause skin irritation (**Anderson et al., 2005: II-2**).
	b. Apply povidone-iodine as per facility guidelines and allow to dry for 30 seconds.	Povidone-iodine has been shown to have similarly high toxicity index to fibroblasts and keratinocyte cells in vitro when compared with CHG and a variety of skin cleansers (**Wilson et al., 2005: II-1**). Most case reports concerning povidone-iodine solutions discuss systemic toxicity involving thyroid function, although cutaneous injury has also been reported (**Sardesai et al, 2011: III**). Povidone-iodine is readily available in single-use applicators. Using a disinfectant in premature infants who weigh less than 1,500 grams and are less than 7 days old carries the risk of skin injury, especially with CHG-containing solutions (**Garland et al., 2009: I**). Solutions with povidone-iodine carry a risk of potential toxicity from iodine absorption in this population (**Khashu et al., 2005: III; Linder et al., 1997: II-3; Mitchell et al., 1991: II-2; Parravicini et al., 1996: II-2; Smerdely et al., 1989: II-2**).
4	Remove all disinfectants as completely as possible with sterile water or saline after the procedure is complete.	Disinfectants should be used with caution on underdeveloped or damaged skin and should always be removed after use on intact skin to prevent tissue damage (**Wilson et al., 2005: II-1**). Chlorhexidine strongly binds to protein in the stratum corneum and can withstand removal even with isopropyl alcohol; thus, it may not be possible to completely remove CHG (**Chapman et al., 2012: III**).
	• Avoid the use of isopropyl alcohol as a primary disinfectant or for removing povidone-iodine or CHG.	Isopropyl alcohol is drying to skin and less efficacious than CHG and povidone-iodine (**Choudhuri et al., 1990: II-1; Maki et al., 1991: I**) and has been associated with chemical burns in premature infants (**Harpin & Rutter, 1982: III; Schick & Milstein, 1981: III**).
5	Use isopropyl alcohol or 2% CHG in isopropyl alcohol for disinfection of needleless connectors and other IV access ports and hubs. a. Scrub the access port for 15–30 seconds. b. Allow the port to dry.	Needleless connectors, access ports, and hubs are sites for potential entry of microorganisms via the intraluminal route of contamination (**Mermel, 2011: III**). These risks may be minimized by scrubbing the access port with an appropriate antiseptic (CHG, povidone-iodine, an iodophor, or 70% isopropyl alcohol) and accessing the port only with sterile devices (**CDC, 2011: III**). A surveillance study of pediatric patients on a bone marrow transplant unit found a dramatic drop in catheter-related bacteremias (from 12 to 3 infections per 1,000 catheter days) after switching from isopropyl alcohol alone to 2% CHG/isopropyl alcohol for catheter connector disinfection; the policy was to provide a 30-second scrub and allow the port to dry completely, but this practice was not audited for compliance (**Soothill et**

al., 2009: II-3). A similar study conducted in infants requiring gastrointestinal surgery and total parenteral nutrition fluids found a high incidence of septicemia (32%), with a decrease in sepsis with coagulase-negative staphylococci and gram-negative bacilli but no reduction in cultures positive with enterococci (**Bishay et al., 2011; II-2**).

Diaper Dermatitis and Diaper Wipes

	Clinical Practice	Referenced Rationale and Quality of Evidence Rating
1	Maintain an optimal skin environment in the perineal area.	Diaper dermatitis is an acute inflammatory reaction of skin in the perineal area (**Heimall, Storey, Steller, & Davis, 2012: III**). Diaper dermatitis typically begins to appear after 1–3 weeks of life (**Atherton, 2004: III; Visscher, Chatterjee, Munson, Bare, & Hoath, 2000: II-3**). Skin care practices such as bathing and emollient use greatly influence the integrity of the skin, which influences its ability to function as a barrier against environmental stresses such as those causing diaper dermatitis (**Atherton, 2001: III**).
	a. Change diapers every 1–3 hours during the day and at least once at night. The genital area should be gently and thoroughly cleansed; avoid rubbing when cleansing the diaper area.	Frequent diaper changes decrease skin wetness and contact with fecal enzymes. Use of absorbent diapers helps maintain skin pH (**Atherton, 2005: III; Berg, Buckingham, & Stewart, 1986: II-2; Campbell, Seymour, Stone, & Milligan, 1987: I; Davis, Leyden, Grove, & Raynor, 1989: I; Neild & Kamat, 2007: III; Shin, 2005: III**). Excessive scrubbing and washing may promote irritation and further damage the barrier properties of the skin surface. Gentle cleansing, rinsing, and patting the area dry is less irritating than rubbing (**Shin, 2005: III; Jackson, 2010: III**). Prolonged contact of skin with a mixture of urine and feces is a primary risk factor for diaper dermatitis. Occlusion of the skin with diapers increases skin wetness and skin surface pH. Some of the bacteria in feces contain ureases (enzymes) that release ammonia from urine, contributing to raising skin pH. Skin wetness increases the susceptibility of the skin to damage from friction. Alkaline skin surface pH increases the activity of skin irritants (fecal proteases and lipases) and hinders the maintenance of a normal skin microflora (**Atherton, 2001: III; Atherton, 2004: III; Atherton, 2005: III; Davies, Dore, & Perissinotto, 2006: I; Lin, Tinkle, & Janniger, 2005: III; Scheinfeld, 2005: III; Stamatas, Zerweck, Grove, & Martin, 2011: II-1; Visscher et al., 2000; II-3**).
	b. Use appropriate methods to cleanse the diaper area. Consider products that have been safety-tested on neonates. Some suggestions include: • soft cloths and water; • soft cloths, water, and a gentle cleanser; and • disposable diaper wipes.	Using water and cotton, a mild soap and water, or baby wipes are methods shown to be adequate in cleansing the newborn buttocks and perianal area (**AAP & ACOG, 2012: III**). Using water alone to cleanse the diaper area may be insufficient to remove feces. Some studies indicate that water and mild cleansers have similar effects on skin parameters such as pH and hydration, while others show that water alone may be more drying. Some cleansers containing emollients may provide further protective effects (**Blume-Peytavi et al., 2009: III**). Infant wipes with a pH buffering capacity have been shown to be well tolerated and more comfortable among infants ages 3–24 months with atopic dermatitis when compared with the use of water only and a wash cloth (**Adam et al., 2009: II-I**). A randomized, controlled trial of 280 full-term infants showed the use of diaper wipes to be equivalent to the use of cotton and water when measuring TEWL, pH, erythema, and skin colonization (**Lavender et al., 2012: I**). Diaper wipes that have been tested on premature infants in the NICU can safely be used for cleansing. A randomized trial of 130 NICU infants com-

Clinical Practice	Referenced Rationale and Quality of Evidence Rating
	paring two types of diaper wipes to cloth and water only found improved diaper area skin condition and barrier function when using diaper wipes made from a soft, nonwoven materials with water and emollient cleansers (**Visscher, Odio, et al., 2009: I**). Some brands of disposable baby wipes contain alcohol, perfumes, or preservatives that may contribute to skin irritation and increase risk for allergic contact dermatitis (**Fields, Nelson, & Powell, 2006: III; Odio, Streicher-Scott, & Hansen, 2001: II-1; Smith & Jacobs, 2009: III**).
c. Consider using super absorbent disposable diapers as an alternative to cloth diapers.	When compared with washable cloth diapers, super absorbent disposable diapers have been associated with a reduced incidence and decreased severity of irritant diaper dermatitis. This finding is likely the result of the quick absorption of urine into the disposable diaper core away from the skin, reducing wetting of the skin and mixing of urine with feces; cloth diapers remain saturated and do not reduce skin wetness in this way (**Atherton, 2005: III; Erasala, Romain, & Merlay, 2011: III; Humphrey, Bergman, & Au, 2006: III**). A number of studies support the use of diapers made with absorbent gel materials, disposable diapers capable of emollient application, and diapers with breathable covers that contribute to decreasing skin wetness and mixing of urine and feces (**Atherton, 2001: III; Atherton, 2004: III; Kosemund et al., 2008: III; Lin et al., 2005: III; Nield & Kamat, 2007: III; Rai et al., 2009: III; Scheinfeld, 2005: III**).
2 Implement strategies to reduce the risk or severity of diaper dermatitis:	Uncomfortable erythema and mild scaling are some of the first signs of diaper dermatitis (**Scheinfeld, 2005: III; Visscher et al., 2000: II-3**). If not appropriately treated, diaper dermatitis can rapidly progress to painful excoriated or ulcerated lesions (**Davies et al., 2006: I; White, Kalus, Caron, & Suski, 2003: III**).
a. Perform a focused skin assessment of the perineal area.	One guideline for the care of diapered/incontinent patients developed at a large pediatric hospital provides a systematic assessment tool and suggested treatment recommendations for diaper dermatitis using six categories (**Heimall et al., 2012: III** [See Appendix B]): • intact skin and no erythema; • intact skin, high risk of breakdown due to causticity of stool, with or without erythema; • intact skin, erythema and no *Candida*; • intact skin, erythema, and evidence of *Candida*; • denuded skin and no *Candida*; • denuded skin with evidence of *Candida*

Clinical Practice	Referenced Rationale and Quality of Evidence Rating
b. Encourage and support breastfeeding through infancy.	The stools of breastfed infants have a lower pH than formula-fed infants and have lower levels of enzymes (proteases, lipases, ureases), resulting in less irritation in the perineal area (**Berg, 1987: III**). Breastfed infants also have a lower urinary pH, which may favorably affect the skin surface pH (**Lin et al., 2005: III**).
c. Use petrolatum-based ointments or skin barriers containing zinc oxide at every diaper change in infants at risk for developing diaper dermatitis. Give preference to formulations that contain fewer additives. Risk factors may include the following: • Frequent stooling • Antibiotic use • Malabsorption • Opiate withdrawal • Abnormal rectal sphincter tone	Risk factors for contact irritant diaper dermatitis include frequent stooling caused by infections, antibiotic use, malabsorption, opiate withdrawal and abnormal rectal sphincter tone (extrophy of the bladder, spina bifida) (**Darmstadt & Dinulos, 2000: III; Davis et al., 1989: I; Lund et al., 1999: III**). The use of consistent prevention strategies, such as the application of topical barriers with every diaper change, can physically block chemical irritants and moisture from contacting the skin and minimize friction, thus significantly reducing the incidence of diaper dermatitis (**Jackson, 2010: III; Noonan, et al., 2006: III**). Because petrolatum provides protection from wetness, a thick layer of petrolatum over the perineal area may prevent skin breakdown (**Heimall et al., 2012: III**). Providing an occlusive barrier can protect the skin from injury and promote wound healing if diaper dermatitis is present (**Atherton, 2005: III; Darmstadt & Dinulos, 2000: III; Ghadially et al., 1992: II-I**). Application of a thick layer of zinc oxide provides a protective barrier that helps prevent further injury while the skin heals (**Lund et al., 1999: III**).
d. Avoid vigorously rubbing the skin barrier product off during cleansing.	Some barriers are thick and stay on the skin after gentle cleansing. It is appropriate to remove only the soiled layer of barrier to avoid vigorous rubbing of skin in the diaper area (**Taquino, 2000: III**).
e. Use alcohol-free skin protectants to provide a barrier between skin and urine or feces in infants more than 28 days old.	Plastic-polymer barrier films that are alcohol-free have been labeled by the FDA as treatment for diaper dermatitis in infants more than 28 days old (**Heimall et al., 2012: III**). Apply these products once every 24 hours.
f. Avoid products containing chemicals that are potentially toxic if absorbed through the skin, such as topical vitamin A.	Diapers, especially when moist, occlude and can compromise the skin barrier, thus increasing the risk of local skin irritation and percutaneous absorption. Some products, such as those containing vitamin A, that are designed to treat diaper dermatitis pose a risk for potential toxicity in neonates, especially those products with multiple active and inactive ingredients. There is insufficient evidence to support the use of topical vitamin A to treat or prevent diaper dermatitis in the newborn. Although percutaneous absorption of retinoic acid (a metabolite of vitamin A) is believed to be minimal, further research is warranted to confirm its safety for use in the neonatal population (**Davies et al., 2006: I**).

	Clinical Practice	Referenced Rationale and Quality of Evidence Rating
3	Treat skin excoriation from contact irritant diaper dermatitis by implementing all of the following methods:	Treatment goals range from the prevention of skin breakdown in an infant with intact skin and no erythema to providing a barrier when there are high risk factors present for skin breakdown and erythema (**Heimall et al., 2012: III**).
	a. Identify and treat the underlying cause.	Malabsorption following acute infectious diarrhea, intestinal resection, or opiate withdrawal may be the underlying causes for significant contact irritant diaper dermatitis. Treatment may include nutritional interventions such as changing to a more elemental diet or use of medications to treat underlying causes such as opiate withdrawal (**Darmstadt & Dinulos, 2000: III; Lund et al., 1999: III**).
	b. Protect injured skin with thick applications of barrier cream or paste, such as zinc oxide. • Consider using an alcohol-free, pectin-based layer covered with petrolatum if zinc oxide alone does not adequately protect the skin from reinjury. • Apply barrier paste or cream in a thick coating. • Cover all skin that may be exposed to irritating agents. • Residual cream should not be removed with diaper changes. • Gently cleanse the area and reapply barrier cream.	Severe diaper dermatitis and excoriated peristomal sites caused by contact with urine, stool, and gastric contents benefit from optimal use of barrier products. Barrier product should be applied in a thick coating. Removing residual cream or paste with diaper changes may cause further damage to the delicate healing tissue (**Taquino, 2000: III**).
	c. Consider oral or topical cholestyramine agents as ordered by the health care provider.	Cholestyramine agents bind to bile acids and help prevent loose stools. These agents work well in infants who excrete high amounts of bile acids in their stools (**White et al., 2003: III**).
4	Identify and treat diaper dermatitis complicated by *Candida albicans* (as evidenced by the presence of red satellite lesions or diagnosed by culture).	*Candida* infection is characterized by the presence of beefy red skin with lesions scattered at the edges (satellite lesions). The skin may or may not need to be denuded (**Heimall et al., 2012: III**).

	Clinical Practice	Referenced Rationale and Quality of Evidence Rating
	a. Apply topical treatment, including antifungal ointments or creams, as ordered. Some antifungal agents include but are not limited to the following: • Nystatin ointment • Clotrimazole ointment • Mupirocin	When candida is present, treatment as well as application of a barrier for the prevention of skin breakdown or further skin breakdown is the goal (**Heimall et al., 2012: III**). Low concentration of antifungal agents in a zinc/petrolatum base has shown to be well tolerated and effective in treating mild-to-severe diaper dermatitis complicated by *Candida* (**Concannon, Gisoldi, Phillips, & Grossman, 2001: I; Spraker et al., 2006: I**). Nystatin ointment is often selected for treatment for diaper dermatitis complicated by *C. albicans*. However, some resistant strains of *Candida* may not respond as well, and another antifungal product may be indicated. In a study of older infants with *Candida* diaper dermatitis, clotrimazole reduced the symptom scores and global assessment more effectively than nystatin ointment; however, both achieved microbiological cure and were safe and well tolerated (**Hoeger, Stark, & Jost, 2010: I**). Mupirocin 2% may also be effective as a topical treatment for diaper dermatitis complicated by *C. albicans*, especially if *Staphylococcus* or *Streptococcus* species are present (**de Wet, Rode, van Dyk, & Millar, 1999: I**).
	b. Treat combination contact irritant and *Candida* diaper dermatitis with a combination of antifungal powder and a barrier as ordered. One suggested protocol is to use the crusting technique, which involves the following: • Apply an antifungal powder. • Seal in the antifungal powder by covering area with a skin protectant. • Apply a thick layer of zinc oxide or petrolatum.	The treatment goal for skin that has both contact irritation and evidence of *Candida* is to prevent further skin breakdown by treating the *Candida* and providing a barrier. This goal can be accomplished using a crusting technique (**Heimall et al., 2012: III**).
5	Use of talcum baby powders or cornstarch is unnecessary and is not recommended to prevent or treat diaper dermatitis in neonates.	Although antifungal powders are useful and safe to treated *Candida* diaper dermatitis, conventional baby powders and cornstarch are not recommended. These powders may exacerbate diaper dermatitis by promoting bacterial and *Candida* growth. Inhaled powder particles can cause respiratory irritation (**Darmstadt & Dinulos, 2000: III; Farrington, 1992: III; Nield & Kamat, 2007: III**).

	Clinical Practice	Referenced Rationale and Quality of Evidence Rating
6	Use of antibiotic ointment is not recommended and is generally unnecessary for routine care of common primary contact irritant diaper dermatitis. When bacterial anal infections are diagnosed, therapy should be initiated under the direction of the health care provider.	Although antibiotic ointments are usually not recommended, one study identified that *S. aureus* was a leading cause of bacterial anal infection, necessitating antimicrobial therapy. Evaluation using cultures and topical and systemic treatments are indicated for this condition (**Heath, Desai, & Silverberg, 2009: III**).
7	Use of topical corticosteroids should be discouraged. If indicated in certain circumstances, this therapy should be implemented under the direction of a health care provider only.	The overuse of topical glucocorticoids to treat diaper dermatitis can lead to the development of Cushing's syndrome, systemic toxicity, and dermal atrophy in infants (**Abraham, 2007: III; Nield & Kamat, 2007: III; Ozon et al., 2007: III**). The greater ratio of surface area to weight during infancy contributes to the much faster rate that infants develop adrenal suppression when compared with adults (**Abraham, 2007: III**).
8	Evaluate the effectiveness of therapeutic interventions and consider allergic contact dermatitis as a potential diagnosis if the response to therapy is not favorable.	There is an increasing prevalence of allergic contact dermatitis in the diaper area because sensitization to allergens is enhanced in the wet environment enclosed by the diaper. This etiology should be considered in patients who are not responsive to the usual therapeutic interventions of frequent diaper changes and emollients (**Smith & Jacob, 2009: III**).
9	Consider using dye-free diapers for allergen avoidance in special circumstances, such as an infant with known allergic contact dermatitis.	The prevalence of allergic reactions to dye in diapers is unknown (**Jackson, 2010: III**). Topically administered corticosteroids are useful in the treatment of allergic contact dermatitis; however, the preferred treatment for diaper dye dermatitis is the use of dye-free diapers for allergen avoidance (**Alberta, Sweeney, & Wiss, 2005: III**).

	Clinical Practice	Referenced Rationale and Quality of Evidence Rating
1	Select and use medical adhesives appropriately to secure life support, monitoring, and other devices in all newborns. • Removal of medical adhesives can cause trauma, such as skin stripping and pain.	Different types of medical adhesives are used in tapes and wound dressings. These include acrylics, hydrocolloids, polyurethanes, hydrogels, silicones, and zinc oxide (**Cutting, 2008: III).** Because of diminished cohesion between the epidermis and dermis (**Holbrook, 1982: III**), even one removal of an adhesive can result in alteration in skin barrier function (**Harpin & Rutter, 1983: II-2; Lund et al., 1997: II-1**). A study including adult volunteers demonstrated an increase in "peel force"—or amount of force needed to remove the adhesive from the skin—has been shown to increase the level of discomfort with adhesive removal (**Dykes & Heggie, 2003: II-2**) and cause trauma, which reduces skin barrier function and increases cutaneous irritancy (**Dykes 2007: II-3**). Some anatomic sites, such as the cheek and back, have a thinner stratum corneum layer and are more vulnerable to skin stripping and disruption of skin barrier function when adhesives are removed (**Breternitz, Flach, Prässler, Elsner, & Fluhr,2007: I**). Adhesives were found to be the primary cause of skin breakdown among infants in the NICU in an evidence-based practice project involving 2,464 neonates (**Lund, Osborne, et al., 2001: II-3**). In one prevalence survey, the incidence of epidermal stripping in pediatric patients reported at a single pediatric hospital was 8% (**Noonan et al., 2006: III**). This prevalence was lower than the 17% reported in a multisite pediatric pressure ulcer and skin breakdown prevalence survey (**McLane et al., 2004: II-2**). The lower rate of epidermal stripping was attributed to the routine use of skin barrier protective films and avoidance of direct tape to skin contact (**Noonan et al., 2006: III**).
2	Choose medical adhesives that cause the least tissue trauma while effectively securing medical devices (such as endotracheal tubes, intravascular catheters, and nasogastric tubes) and monitoring equipment, as well as wound dressings. The choices include the following:	Some adhesives have been shown to cause less tissue trauma in studies comparing different products (**Cutting, 2008: III; Dykes, 2007: II-3; Morris, Emsley, Marland, Meuleneire, & White, 2009: II-3**). Other considerations include how well the adhesive functions, such as how well it adheres when there is exudate or moisture, how it protects from these, and how it functions as a barrier (**Taquino, 2000: III**).
	a. Acrylics	A single application of plastic, perforated acrylic tape resulted in disruption of skin barrier function in neonates ranging from 25–42 weeks of age (**Lund et al., 1997: II-1**). Yet these types of adhesives adhere effectively to skin and medical devices and are commonly used in intensive care settings.
	b. Hydrocolloids	Hydrocolloids have been shown to cause skin trauma equal to acrylic tape when removed at 24 hours (**Lund et al., 1997: II-1**). Other studies also report decreased skin barrier function, seen with increased TEWL and erythema under hydrocolloids (**Zilmer, Agren, Gottrup, & Karlsmark, 2006: II-3**). However, these barriers are still used because they absorb

Clinical Practice	Referenced Rationale and Quality of Evidence Rating
	moisture, mold well to skin surfaces, and serve as a platform for other adhesives (**Lund & Tucker, 2003: III**).
c. Hydrogels	Hydrogel adhesives should not be used when adherence is critical, as the adhesive product may dislodge (**Lund et al., 1997: II-1**). Use of hydrogel adhesives can reduce the trauma associated with electrode removal (**Darmstadt & Dinulos, 2000: III; Lund et al., 1997: II-1; Webster & McCosker, 1994: I**). Use of limb electrodes leaves the chest wall free of devices and permits easier access for auscultation and assessment (**Malloy & Perez-Woods, 1991: III**).
d. Polyurethanes	Polyurethanes, such as transparent adhesive dressings, allow visualization of catheter insertions sites and are permeable to water vapor, oxygen, and carbon dioxide, allowing the skin to breathe (**Darmstadt & Dinulos, 2000: III; Lund & Kuller, 2007: III**). Polyurethanes are commonly used as dressings for intravascular devices, such as central venous catheters.
e. Silicones	Silicone-based adhesive products have been shown to improve adherence to wounds and reduce discomfort to patients with adhesive removal. This technology holds promise for developing products that adhere and cause minimal trauma when removed from neonatal skin (**Dykes & Heggie, 2003: II-2; Dykes, 2007: II-3; Dykes, Heggie, & Hill, 2001: II-1; Morris et al., 2009: II-3**). However, silicone adhesives do not adhere well to plastic devices, such as nasogastric tubes and cannulas, which may limit their use for attaching some medical devices.
f. Zinc oxide adhesives	Zinc oxide adhesives have been shown to significantly reduce skin barrier function, resulting in increased TEWL, compared with a hydrocolloid adhesive (**Nielsen et al., 2005: II-2**).
3 Consider protecting the skin from medical adhesives with silicone-based skin protective films.	Skin barrier films have been shown to protect the skin from adhesives, as well as fecal and ostomy output and urine. However, these protective films can be irritants to skin and require removal with solvents, which can also irritate the skin. Some also contained benzyl alcohol, which should be avoided in neonates (**Black, 2007: III**). Silicone-based skin barrier films do not sting when applied, rapidly evaporate, and do not leave a residue. In addition to the general benefits of silicone-based skin protectants in neonates (**Irving, 2001: III**), one study of premature infants showed both skin protection and the additional benefit of reduced TEWL (**Brandon et al., 2010: I**).

	Clinical Practice	Referenced Rationale and Quality of Evidence Rating
4	Remove medical adhesives slowly and carefully using moistened gauze or saline pledgets.	There are three categories of adhesive removers: alcohol/organic-based solvents, oil-based solvents, and silicone-based removers (**Black, 2007: III**).
	a. Pull medical adhesive tapes on a horizontal plane, folding the tape back onto itself while continuously wetting the adhesive-skin interface.	A technique involving slowly pulling adhesives at a very low angle, parallel to the skin surface, while holding the surrounding skin in place, may reduce epidermal stripping (**Lund & Tucker, 2003: III**).
	b. Alternatively, use mineral oil or petrolatum to loosen tape unless retaping is necessary at the site.	Mineral oil or petrolatum leaves an oily residue that may prevent the next adhesive appliance from attaching properly (**Lund & Kuller, 2007: III**).
	c. Consider the use of silicone-based adhesive remover when applicable.	Silicone-based removers form an interposing layer between adhesive and skin, evaporate readily after application, do not leave a residue, and are inert, reducing the risk of toxicity (**Black, 2007: III**). The use of silicone-based removers has been advocated for patients with extremely fragile skin, such as infants with epidermolysis bullosa (**Stephen-Haynes, 2008: III**).
5	Avoid using the following products whenever possible:	
	a. Alcohol/organic-based products	Alcohol/organic-based products dissolve the adhesive components. They evaporate readily and do not leave a residue (**Black, 2007: III**), but insufficient evidence exists to demonstrate the safety of these solvents, as they contain hydrocarbon derivatives or petroleum distillates that have potential or proven toxicity. The potential risk of absorption and toxicity is greater in premature babies because of their immature stratum corneum and in newborns because of their large surface-area-to-body-weight ratio. One case report described a severe skin reaction to an adhesive remover applied to a premature infant (**Ittman & Bozynski, 1993: III**).
	b. Oil-based solvents	Oil-based solvents release the bond between skin and adhesive and are based on paraffin or citrus oil extracts. However, these do not evaporate when applied, leave a residual on the skin similar to mineral oil or petrolatum, and can potentially be absorbed, with unknown effects (**Black, 2007: III**).
	c. Enhancing bonding agents	The bond between adhesive and epidermis is stronger than the fragile cohesion between epidermis and dermis in premature infants (**Holbrook, 1982: III**); epidermal stripping may result when adhesives are removed. Tincture of benzoin, when used in adults, is drying to skin, can cause irritation, and can occlude the skin and impair its function (**Gill, 1982: III; Weber et al., 1987: III**).

Clinical Practice	Referenced Rationale and Quality of Evidence Rating
d. Adhesive bandages after drawing laboratory samples	Application of adhesives should be avoided whenever possible. Pressure with a cotton ball may be sufficient to stop bleeding (**Gordon & Montgomery, 1996: III**).
6 Observe for morbidity associated with medical adhesive use in very-low-birthweight infants, such as anetoderma of prematurity.	Anetoderma is defined as atrophic patches of skin caused by dermal thinning. A series of nine infants, 24–29 weeks of gestation, were noted to have atrophic skin lesions, located on the abdomen, chest, upper arms, and thighs, associated with placement of monitoring leads or temperature probes (**Goujon et al., 2010: III; Prizant, Lucky, Frieden, Burton, & Suarez, 1996: II-2**).

Emollients

	Clinical Practice	Referenced Rationale and Quality of Evidence Rating
1	Emollients may be used to restore integrity to dry or cracking skin.	Emollients protect the integrity of the stratum corneum and enhance barrier function (**Ghadially et al., 1992: II-1; Kiechl-Kohlendorfer, Berger, & Inzinger, 2008: I; Lane & Drost, 1993: I**).
	a. At the first sign of dryness, fissures, or flaking, apply an emollient every 12 hours or as needed.	Emollients can reduce or treat dry scaly skin, cracking, or fissures on skin surfaces (**Blume-Peytavi et al., 2009: III; Ghadially et al., 1992: II-1; Lane & Drost, 1993: I**).
	b. Apply emollient gently to skin, especially with very-low-birthweight neonates, to avoid friction.	Friction may cause skin irritation and breakdown, especially in very-low-birthweight babies (**Darmstadt & Dinulos, 2000: III**).
	c. Observe for development of systemic infections, such as coagulase-negative *Staphylococcus* infections, especially in neonates weighing less than 750 grams.	While the use of emollients is effective in treating dry or cracked skin, a Cochrane review of four randomized, controlled studies found that prophylactic emollient use for the first 2 weeks of life is associated with an increased risk of coagulase-negative *Staphylococcus epidermidis* infection (**Conner, Soll, & Edwards, 2003: I**). Other studies examining the prophylactic use of emollients have not found higher infection rates when comparing emollient therapy with no treatment (**Beeram et al., 2006: II-2; Kiechl-Kohlendorfer et al., 2008: I**) or with alcohol-free skin protectants (**Brandon et al., 2010: I**). The benefits of emollient use for prevention of dermatitis and skin breakdown should be weighed against the risk of infection.
2	Emollients should be provided in unit dose or patient-specific containers. Every effort should be made to maintain sterility of the emollient container. All surrounding treatment surfaces that may be contaminated by emollients should be thoroughly cleaned.	Contamination of surfaces and emollient containers should be avoided to prevent infections (**Campbell, Zaccaria, & Baker, 2000: II-3; Darmstadt & Dinulos, 2000: III**).
3	Emollients may interfere with adherence of adhesives.	Skin residues can interfere with adhesion of adhesives (**Kiechl-Kohlendorfer et al., 2008: I; Lund & Tucker, 2003: III**). Preservative-free, water-miscible, petrolatum-based emollients can be removed with soap and water if necessary (**Nopper et al., 1996: I**).
4	Emollients may be used to treat discrete areas of skin dryness, flaking, or fissures for infants on radiant warming tables or receiving phototherapy.	There is little evidence of increased hyperthermia or tissue burns when emollients are used for infants on radiant warming tables or under phototherapy lights (**Darmstadt & Dinulos, 2000: III; Nopper et al., 1996: I**). Transepidermal water loss was reduced when a clear topical ointment was used on jaundiced preterm infants under phototherapy (**Wananukul, Praisuwanna, & Kesorncam, 2001; II-2**).

	Clinical Practice	Referenced Rationale and Quality of Evidence Rating
5	Routine emollient use may be indicated in healthy, full-term newborns with "cradle cap" or atopic dermatitis (eczema).	Cradle cap, also known as infant seborrheic dermatitis, is a condition in which thick, crusty, yellow scales occur on the scalp and sometimes the face, neck, or behind the ears. Unlike atopic dermatitis, it is not itchy or uncomfortable. The cause may be increased sebum production from maternal hormones, although the lipophilic yeast, *Malassezia furfur*, may also be involved. Treatment involves applying a moisturizer or oil to the affected area and leaving it on for an hour or longer, washing with a gentle baby shampoo, then moisturizing again. If this treatment is not effective, consultation with a health professional is advised, as antifungal agents or medicated shampoos may be indicated (**Smoker, 2007: III**). In the case of atopic dermatitis, the "soak and seal" approach to bathing and moisturizing is recommended. This involves bathing the baby daily using a moisturizing liquid cleanser, followed by an emollient application to all affected skin. These recommendations may also be beneficial for infants at risk for developing atopic dermatitis because of a strong family history for this disease (either parent or sibling with atopic dermatitis) (**Bieber, 2010: III; Blume-Peytavi et al., 2009: III**).
	Special Needs for Developing Countries	
1	Because of differences in mechanisms of transmission of transcutaneous sepsis and resources available, one or both of the following approaches may be appropriate:	In developing countries, environmental contamination may lead to microscopic invasion of organisms through the skin leading to sepsis (**Darmstadt, Saha, et al., 2007: I**), rather than through the insertion sites of medical devices, which are used less often in developing countries (**Polin et al., 2012: III**). Significant differences may exist in resource availability, environmental cleanliness, bacteriologic profile, and social customs in some developing countries (**Ahmadpour-Kacho et al., 2006: I**).
	a. Linoleate-enriched oils might increase skin barrier function.	Vegetable oils high in linoleic acid, applied topically, may provide a low-cost, simple alternative for enhancing epidermal barrier function, decreasing the risk of infection and hypothermia, and improving survival of premature infants or those with malnutrition (**Darmstadt et al., 2004: I; Darmstadt et al., 2005: I; Darmstadt et al., 2008: I**).
	b. Topical treatment with various types of oils is a common practice in some cultures.	The type of oil used should be evaluated. Mustard and olive oils, commonly used in some developing countries, have been shown to increase TEWL and reduce skin barrier function, while sunflower seed and safflower oils reduce TEWL and improve skin barrier function (**Darmstadt & Saha, 2002: II-2**). Use of more effective products, such as sunflower or manufactured emollients, may be more acceptable to parents (**Ahmed et al., 2007: III**) but are based upon their availability and cost (**Ahmed et al., 2007: III; LeFevre et al., 2010: I**).

Transepidermal Water Loss

	Clinical Practice	Referenced Rationale and Quality of Evidence Rating
1	Use a single technique or combination of techniques to reduce TEWL and minimize evaporative heat loss in premature infants less than 30 weeks of gestation.	Premature infants of less than 30 weeks of gestation have an immature stratum corneum that allows TEWL as well as evaporative heat loss (**Fluhr et al., 2010: III; Hammarlund & Sedin, 1979: II-2; Harpin & Rutter, 1985: II-2**). Premature infants of 23–25 weeks of gestation may have TEWL 10 times higher than term infants (**Agren et al., 1998: II-3**). Infants of less than 24 weeks of gestation tend to have higher insensible water loss (50–60 mL/kg/d) during the first 5 days of life despite the use of highly humidified incubators (**Wada, Kusuda, Takahashi, & Nishida, 2008: III**). Premature infants do not have mature skin barrier function until 30–32 weeks post-conceptional age (**Fluhr et al., 2010: III; Kalia et al., 1998: II-2**). The long-term detrimental effects of uncontrolled TEWL have not been studied prospectively in terms of neonatal morbidity and length of hospital stay, but retrospective studies suggest there may be an association (**Bhandari et al., 2005: II-2**). If methods to prevent excessive TEWL are not employed, increased fluid intake may be needed to replace fluid loss from the skin and prevent dehydration, hypernatremia, and energy loss (**Agren et al., 1998: II-3; Bhatia, 2006: III; Sedin et al., 1985: III; Wada et al., 2008: III**).
2	Choose one or more of the following techniques to reduce TEWL:	There is limited research comparing outcomes of various treatment modalities.
	a. To reduce postnatal temperature decreases caused by excessive evaporative heat loss, place the neonate in an occlusive polyethylene bag or wrap from the shoulders down without drying the infant's body while the infant is under a radiant heater. Remove the wrapping after the infant has been stabilized in the delivery room and admitted to the NICU. Monitor temperature frequently during use.	Polyethylene wrap applied immediately after birth reduces the postnatal fall in temperature in premature infants less than 28 weeks of gestation more effectively than conventional drying using radiant warmers for stabilization in the delivery room (**Bissinger & Annibale, 2010: III; Knobel et al., 2005: I; Vohra, Frent, Campbell, Abbott, & Whyte, 1999: I; Vohra et al., 2004: I**). A higher ambient temperature in the delivery room is also beneficial to maintaining temperature, with or without the bag (**Knobel et al., 2005: I**). Current AAP Neonatal Resuscitation Program guidelines suggest the use of polyurethane bags in the initial stabilization of premature infants less than 29 weeks of gestation (**AAP & American Heart Association, 2010: III**). Monitor temperature closely for hyperthermia (**McCall, Alderdice, Halliday, Jemkin & Vohra, 2010: III**). A controlled study using a thermal sweating mannequin concluded that use of polyethylene bag reduces total heat loss by 30–40%, primarily through reduction of evaporative water loss (**Belghazi et al., 2006: II-1**).

b. Provide humidity at levels of more than 70% relative humidity for the first 7 days of life.

Transepidermal water loss in extremely-low-birthweight infants at 25–26 weeks of gestation is reduced by half when the relative humidity is increased from 20% to 60% (**Hammarlund & Sedin, 1979: II-2**). High humidity reduces TEWL and evaporative heat loss, resulting in improved temperature stability (**Hammarlund & Sedin, 1979: II-2; Harpin & Rutter, 1985: II-2**). Incubator humidity practices continue to vary depending on providers' perceptions of benefits, which include decreased TEWL, improved fluid and electrolyte balance, and risk of infection (**Sinclair, Crisp & Sinn, 2009: III**).

High humidity has been shown to reduce fluid requirements and improve electrolyte balance in premature infants when compared with historical control groups (**Bhatia, 2006: III; Gaylord et al., 2001: II-2; Kim et al., 2010: II-2**). However, humidity levels above 90% and water condensation inside of incubators may reduce irradiance levels in blue LED phototherapy and halogen spot phototherapy, thus decreasing effectiveness of these therapies (**De Carvalho, Torrao, & Moreira, 2011: II-3**).

A polyethylene tent with a constant humidity flow heated to body temperature prevented excess TEWL and improved temperature control in premature infants who were cared for on a radiant warmer. This humidity control method was also found to be efficient for initial warming of an infant at birth (**Meyer, Payton, Salmon, Hutchinson, & de Klerk, 2001: II-2**).

c. Use servo-controlled humidification systems in incubators that actively heat and evaporate water separately from circulating heat, rather than the passive "tray" type of humidification.
   - Clean incubator humidity trays per facility protocol and manufacturer instructions.

Servo-controlled, actively generated humidification systems do not cause airborne aerosols that can be contaminated with microorganisms; they can be set for precise control of humidity levels and allow humidity levels to recover more rapidly because of continually added heated water vapor (**Drucker & Marshall, 1995: III; Marshall, 1997: III**). Incubator humidity chambers must be accessible for proper cleaning and should be cleaned on a regular schedule or as needed to prevent spread of infection (**Etienne et al., 2011: III**).

d. After the first week of life, gradually decrease relative humidity to 50% until the infant is 28 days old.
   - Consider continuing 50% humidity until 30–32 weeks postconceptional age.

In extremely-low-birthweight infants, TEWL usually drops by 50% after 7 days of life. Serum sodium and fluid balance are generally normalized by the first week of life. Infants in an environment where humidity was decreased to 50% after 7 days in 85% humidity appeared to have better skin barrier maturation at 28 days of life and did not have increased dehydration or hyponatremia when compared with infants cared for in 75% humidity for the first month (**Agren, Sjors, & Sedin, 2006: I; Kim et al., 2010: II-2**). Infants born at less than 26 weeks of gestation may require 50% humidity past 28 days of life (**Fluhr et al., 2010: III**) because they do not have mature skin barrier function until 30–32 weeks postconceptional age (**Kalia et al., 1998: II-2**).

Clinical Practice	Referenced Rationale and Quality of Evidence Rating
e. Choose a thermoregulation device on the basis of individual facility protocol and availability.	Both radiant warmers and dry incubators (no added humidity) reduce humidity when heating because of a reduction in ambient water vapor pressure, although the effect is generally found to be more significant under radiant heat (**Kjartansson, Arsan, Hammarlund, Sjors, & Sedin, 1995: II-1**). Radiant heat and dry incubators equally increase TEWL in premature infants of 27–34 weeks of gestation (**Maayan-Metzger, Yosipovitch, Hadad, & Sirota, 2004: II-1**). Three small studies comparing single- and double-walled incubators found decreased temperature loss, decreased heat production, and decreased radiant heat loss with the use of double-walled incubators (**Laroia, Phelps, & Roy, 2007: II-1**).
f. Use supplemental conductive heat from water-filled pads or heated mattresses to reduce heater output from radiant warmers.	Supplemental conductive heat reduces radiant heater output and may result in less drying of the surrounding air (**Topper & Stewart, 1984: II-1**). Newer models of radiant warmers have warm, gelled mattresses that provide supplemental conductive heat up to 38.5°C (101.3°F).
g. Use polyethylene coverings to reduce TEWL and evaporative heat loss if unable to provide a humidified environment for procedures. Plastic wraps should not be in contact with skin surfaces for prolonged periods.	Polyethylene is preferred over polystyrene and other plastic materials because it transmits long-wavelength radiant energy (**LeBlanc, 1991: III**). Occlusive plastic wraps in contact with skin surfaces may cause maceration of the skin and result in breakdown (**Aly, Shirley, Cunico, & Maibach, 1978: II-1**).
h. Consider the use of topical treatments, including but not limited to the following:	
• Semipermeable transparent adhesive dressings applied to the back and abdomen to reduce TEWL.	Transparent adhesive dressings can reduce TEWL by as much as 50% (**Bustamante & Steslow, 1989: I; Knauth, Gordin, McNelis, & Baumgart, 1989: II-1; Mancini et al., 1994: II-1; Vernon, Lane, Wischerath, Davis, & Menegus, 1990: II-1**). A prospective study found no difference in fluid intake or serum sodium levels in infants treated with transparent dressings compared with those who did not have the dressings, although skin condition appeared better in infants with covered skin (**Donahue et al., 1996: I**). A retrospective study reported that semipermeable transparent dressings did significantly improve fluid and sodium balance, as well as improving weight gain and survival and decreasing the incidence of bronchopulmonary dysplasia (**Bhandari et al., 2005: II-2**). The deleterious effect of removing transparent adhesive dressings on skin barrier function is similar to that of other adhesives (**Lund et al., 1997: II-1**) and is a consideration for clinical use.

Clinical Practice	Referenced Rationale and Quality of Evidence Rating
• Sterile topical ointment	In a study of 54 infants at 27 weeks of gestation or less, those receiving emollient therapy during the first 2 weeks of life had significantly better urine output and required less IV fluids to maintain homeostasis than those who were not treated with topical emollients (**Beeram et al., 2006: II-2**).
• Alcohol-free skin protectant	A randomized, controlled study of 69 premature infants born before 33 weeks of gestation found that alcohol-free skin protectants were as effective as emollients in decreasing TEWL (**Brandon et al., 2010: I**).
3 Consider the effect of various phototherapy devices on TEWL.	Halogen (spotlight) phototherapy increases TEWL as much as 20% (**Grunhagen, De Boer, De Beaufort, & Walther, 2001: II-2; Mayaan-Metzger, Yosipovitch, Hadad, & Sirota, 2001: II-2**) and results in significantly higher TEWL than conventional phototherapy (**Dani et al., 2001: I**). Fluorescent (banklight) phototherapy has not been shown to increase TEWL (**Kjartansson, Hammarlund, & Sedin 1992: II-2).** LED phototherapy lights do not increase TEWL (**Bertini et al., 2008: I**). Transepidermal water loss reduction strategies, such as use of emollients and high humidity, have been shown to be effective and safe during phototherapy (**Dani et al., 2001: I; Wananukul & Praisuwanna, 2002: I**).

Skin Breakdown

	Clinical Practice	Referenced Rationale and Quality of Evidence Rating
1	Identify risk factors for skin injury for each infant. Risk factors may include but are not limited to the following: • Gestational age less than 32 weeks • Edema • Dehydration • Immobility due to illness, medications • Use of vasopressors • Use of endotracheal tubes, nasogastric or orogastric tubes, vascular access devices, monitors, electrodes, or probes • Surgical wound • Ostomies • Nasal CPAP • High-frequency ventilators • ECMO • Prolonged EEG monitoring	The AWHONN/NANN RBP4 identified a series of items with potential for skin injury (**Lund, Osborne, et al., 2001: II-3**). Patients on respiratory support, particularly high-frequency ventilation (which makes regular turning and repositioning difficult) and NCPAP, and infants with significant perfusion alterations are the most at risk for pressure ulcers and should be carefully assessed during hospitalization, particularly in the area of the head, nares, and ears (**Fujii, Sugama, Okuwa, Sanada, & Mizokami, 2010: II-2; McLane et al., 2004: II-2; Reddy, Kogan, & Glick, 2011: III; Schindler et al., 2011: II-3**). Patients on continuous EEG monitoring are also at risk for skin injury (**Jarrar, Buchhalter, Williams, McKay, & Luketich, 2011: II-3**).
2	Provide adequate nutritional support for all infants.	Nutrition plays an important role in prevention of skin breakdown and wound healing and should be assessed and individualized for every patient (**Stotts, 2007: III; Taquino, 2000: III**). Nutritional care for neonates should include adequate fluid, calories, and nutritional components, such as amino acids, proteins, carbohydrates, fats, vitamins, and trace minerals. Premature infants have greater nutritional requirements than term infants because of their diminished nutrient stores at birth (**Ditzenberger, 2010: III**).
3	Prevent or minimize the risk of skin breakdown by using one or more of the following methods:	The epidermal barrier, the top layer of the skin, is the body's first line of defense; cutaneous injury compromises this protection. In two prospective observational studies of iatrogenic complications in NICU patients, cutaneous injury in neonates is highest among infants less than 27 weeks of gestation, although the skin injury is generally minor (**Kugelman et al., 2008: II-3; Ligi, Arnaud, Jouve, Tardieu, Sambuc, & Simeoni, 2008: II-3**).
	a. Assess skin under medical devices frequently (every 1–4 hours) to identify pressure points secondary to medical device use.	Many pressure ulcers can be prevented with routine observation and monitoring of the skin under medical devices such as nasal CPAP prongs and masks, IV catheter hubs, arm boards, trachesotomy tubes, and plaster cast edges. Routine rotation of devices such as blood pressure cuffs, pulse

	Clinical Practice	Referenced Rationale and Quality of Evidence Rating
		oximetry probes, temperature probes and continuous EEG recordings is also necessary to prevent pressure ulcers (**Baharestani , 2007: III**).
	b. Use products to prevent skin surface breakdown, such as alcohol-free skin protectants, or devices that help prevent pressure ulcers, such as protective padding, water mattresses, air mattresses, gelled mattresses, and blanket-covered sheepskin, whenever possible.	Extremely-low-birthweight infants are at highest risk for skin breakdown because of skin immaturity (**Brandon et al., 2010: I; Kugelman et al., 2008: II-3**). Infants at risk for pressure ulcers include those on high-frequency ventilation and ECMO life support because they are more difficult to turn or move. Pressure ulcers from NCPAP may occur from inadequate monitoring or inappropriate applications or size of the nasal prongs, mask, or head-securing devices (**Sardesai et al., 2011: III**). Nasal ulcers due to NCPAP use accounted for 50% of the pressure ulcers seen in NICU patients (**Fujii et al., 2010: II-2**). In a prospective evaluation of 989 neonates, the incidence of nasal trauma due to nasal CPAP was as high as 42.5%; this study used a standardized system to describe the degree of injury, and most were considered mild (**Fischer et al., 2010: II-2**). Hypotension leading to peripheral tissue hypoperfusion may also be a risk factor for skin breakdown. Common sites for pressure ulcers include the occiput of the head, nares, and ears. Other infants at risk include those who must remain immobile for prolonged periods of time, such as following surgery for bladder extrophy or tracheal surgery (**Darmstadt & Dinulos, 2000: III; Fox, 2011: III; Harris et al., 2003: III; Sardesai et al., 2011: III; Schindler et al., 2011: II-3**).
	c. Petrolatum or petrolatum-based ointments protect from moisture in the perineal area. Alcohol-free skin protectants can also be used for this purpose and to protect from adhesive-related injury.	Very-low-birthweight infants have an underdeveloped stratum corneum that is more susceptible to injuries caused by moisture and adhesive removal (**Baharestani, 2007: III; Brandon et al., 2010: I; Darmstadt & Dinulos, 2000: III**). Refer to the section “Medical Adhesives” in this Guideline.
4	Determine the potential cause of skin breakdown to help guide treatment: • Adhesive removal • Burn/thermal/chemical injury • Abrasion/friction • Diaper dermatitis • Pressure ulcer • Infection • Heel stick	The cause of skin breakdown will often determine the optimal treatment regimen and may lead to strategies to prevent further disruption (**Lund et al., 1999: III**).

Clinical Practice	Referenced Rationale and Quality of Evidence Rating
5 Assess the wound stage of skin breakdown: a. Hemostasis b. Inflammation c. Proliferation and repair d. Maturation and remodeling	Wound-healing occurs in a cascade of events beginning with hemostasis and ending with maturation and remodeling. After bleeding is controlled, the inflammatory stage begins the process of removing the damaged tissue and debris. Decreased function of macrophages, such as with the use of corticosteroids, will hinder healing and prolong the inflammatory stage. New tissue is formed during the proliferation and repair stage. During this stage, the skin is covered with epidermis. The maturation and remodeling stage continues for 12–18 months, during which time the new skin and tissue remain vulnerable to reinjury (**Fox, 2011: III**).
6 Treat skin breakdown and excoriations using one or more of the following methods:	There is little clinically researched information comparing wound care products among neonates. Understanding the principles of moist wound healing, gentle cleansing and prevention of mechanical trauma, and choosing and properly applying the appropriate dressing will lead to better outcomes for neonatal wounds (**Bolton, 2004: III; Fox, 2011: III; Taquino, 2000: III**). Specific wound management strategies should be matched to the stage of wound healing, the amount of wound moisture, and the presence of eschar or infection (**Fox, 2011: III; Rolstad & Ovington, 2007: III**).
a. Obtain skin cultures, Gram stains, and potassium hydroxide preparations from wounds that show signs of infection, such as edema, warmth, pain, excess erythema, the presence of vesicles, pustules, or widespread erythematous rash, as ordered by the primary health care provider.	Identifying the pathogen allows for appropriate antimicrobial therapy. Cutaneous manifestations can precede systemic bacterial or fungal disease, and Candida dermatitis is recognized as an early presentation of invasive fungal disease in the extremely-low-birthweight infant (**Benjamin et al., 2010: II-2**). Colonization of the skin by coagulase-negative Staphylococcus occurs after birth, but systemic infection requires disruption of the epidermal barrier (**Dinulos & Pace, 2008: III**). Therefore, all wounds are considered colonized, but not all wounds are infected. The stimulatory effect of bacteria on wound healing has long been recognized. Bacteria that colonize the wound are believed to help initiate the inflammatory or first stage of wound healing (**Fox, 2011: III; Mendenhall & Eichenfield, 2000: III; Scemons & Elston, 2009: III**). However, if a wound goes beyond colonization and becomes infected, this process prolongs the inflammatory process and delays wound healing (**Fox, 2011: III**).
b. Cleanse the affected area using body-temperature normal saline diluted 1:1 with sterile water or undiluted normal saline with each dressing change. • A 20–60-mL syringe with a blunt needle or IV catheter can be used to gently debride the area of exudate.	The object of wound cleansing is to break the bond between tissue and particles of foreign debris, bacteria, or dirt and to assist in the removal of necrotic tissue. Necrotic tissue will impede wound healing, and removal is important to reduce the level of bacterial contamination (**Jones, 2000: III; Rolstad & Ovington, 2007: III; Taquino, 2000: III**). Mechanical trauma to the wound can occur from overzealous attempts to cleanse it by scrubbing (**Rodeaver, 1989: III**). Avoid the use of antiseptic skin cleansers such as hydrogen peroxide, povidone-iodine, iodophor, Dakin's solution, acetic acid, and any alcohol-containing antiseptic, even diluted. In vitro studies have shown they can cause injury to delicate or healing tissue, are toxic to cells, and may actually delay the healing process (**Lineaweaver et al., 1985:**

II-1; Rolstad & Ovington, 2007: III; Taquino, 2000: III; Wilson et al., 2005: II-1).

c. Antifungal ointment can be used for fungal infections. Systemic treatment may be indicated for very-low-birthweight infants who have temperature instability, lethargy, hypotension, thrombocytopenia, or a positive skin culture for yeast and whose respiratory status is unstable.

Infants most likely to develop fungal sepsis are extremely premature infants with the following additional risk factors: have a central venous line or endotracheal tube, have had abdominal surgery, or are receiving broad-spectrum antibiotics or a prolonged course of postnatal steroids (**Devlin, 2006: III**). Although the most common organism seen is *C. albicans*, deep fungal infection with *Aspergillosis, Rhizopus*, and *Fusarium* have also been reported and often arise at sites of tape occlusion (**Smolinski et al., 2005**); a biopsy is sometimes necessary to diagnose these infections (**Hook & Eichenfield, 2011: III**).

Congenital cutaneous infection appears as a generalized rash in term newborns. In premature infants, it presents with vesicles, pustules, or widespread erythematous rash. Cutaneous manifestations of candidiasis infections (thrush, diaper dermatitis, or burn-like dermatitis) often precede positive blood cultures. Early treatment, both topical and systemic, can prevent devastating disseminated fungal disease (**Darmstadt, Dinulos, & Miller, 2000: III; Kaufman, 2003: III**). Most candidiasis species found in the NICU are sensitive to fluconazole and amphotericin B (**Devlin, 2006: III**). Oral thrush is most commonly treated with an oral antifungal preparation such as nystatin (**Witt, 2004: III**).

d. If extensive bacterial colonization is suspected, antibiotic ointment may be used sparingly every 8–12 hours.

While some antibiotic ointments are useful in treating gram-positive organisms, they may promote growth of gram-negative organisms. Polymyxin, or neomycin, is not recommended because of its potential for subsequent sensitization (**Smack et al., 1996: I**). Triple antibiotic preparations and neomycin cause contact sensitivity in about 15% of cases and may result in substantial absorption when applied to large denuded areas (**Cisler-Cahill, 2006: III**). Sensitization to bacitracin has also been reported with increasing frequency (**Marks et al., 1995: II-2**).

Skin infection with MRSA has been reported, typically during the second week of life. Often, pustular vesicles appear in the groin or perineum as the initial finding. Infection occurs more often in male infants and those born via cesarean delivery (**Carey & Long, 2010: III**).

Vancomycin remains a reliable therapy for systemic treatment of MRSA. Both mupirocin nasal and mupirocin ointment are used for the treatment of MRSA colonization. Mupirocin nasal was found to eradicate nasal colonization in pediatric patients, and the FDA has approved it for use in patients over 2 months of age; use in younger patients is considered an off-label use (**Neofax, 2011**).

e. Petrolatum-based ointments can be used on uninfected or infected lesions after

Petrolatum has been shown to improve healing, reduce skin growth of gram-negative organisms, and decrease the severity of dermatitis (**Ghadially et al., 1992: II-1; Nopper et al., 1996: I; Smack et al., 1996: I**).

cleansing and application of antibacterial ointment. Do not use on fungal lesions.

An association between petrolatum emollients used twice daily for the first 2 weeks of life and coagulase-negative *S. epidermidis* infection has been demonstrated in a subset of infants weighing less than 750 grams in a multisite, randomized, controlled trial involving 1,191 premature infants weighing less than 1,000 grams; there were no differences in gram-negative bacterial or fungal infections between the prophylactic emollient and control group (**Edwards, Conner, & Soll, 2004: I**). The benefits of emollient use for prevention of dermatitis and skin breakdown should be weighed against the risk of infection. In this randomized trial, emollients were used to treat skin dryness in the control infants without significant increases in infection rates (**Edwards et al., 2004: I**).

f. Use silicone-based adhesive dressings, hydrocolloid, polyurethane film, or hydrogel dressings for wounds or large denuded areas.

An appropriate dressing will be occlusive and nonadherent, provide moist healing that promotes rapid migration of epithelial cells, and protect the wound from further injury or trauma (**Lund et al., 1999: III; Taquino, 2000: III**).

Silicone-based adhesive dressings have been shown to improve adherence to wounds and reduce trauma and discomfort to patients with removal (**Dykes et al., 2001: II-1; Gotschall, Morrison, & Eichelberger, 1998: I; Morris et al., 2009: II-3**). These products can be used in conjunction with hydrogel dressings, antimicrobial topical agents, or petrolatum ointment.

Hydrocolloid dressings absorb exudate and create a moist, acidic environment that aids in the removal of necrotic tissue, while the outer layer is waterproof and acts as a barrier (**Irving, 1999: III; Sawatzky-Dicksson & Bodnaryk, 2006: III**).

Hydrogels consist of 80–90% water, which makes them soothing and gentle to the skin while keeping the wound moist (**Cisler-Cahill, 2006: III**). Hydrogels facilitate autodebridement of the wound by rehydrating sloughing tissue and enhancing the rate of autolysis. Two forms of hydrogels are currently available: amorphous gel and sheet dressings. The choice of products is based on the type and site of the wound and fluid-handling capacity needed. Several articles report good wound healing using various forms of hydrogel: sheet dressing (**Cisler-Cahill, 2006: III**), gel (**Lehr, Luli-Butica, Lindblad, Kazzi, & Aranda, 2004: II-3**), and gel over the wound enclosed in a polythene bag, forming a glove or boot (**Thomas, Rowe, Keats, & Morgan, 1997: II-3**).

Transparent adhesive dressings increase cellular proliferation associated with improved barrier function without increasing bacterial or fungal colonization on intact skin (**Mancini et al., 1994: II-1**). They are vapor- and moisture-porous but impervious to bacteria and other particles. Polyurethane film dressings lack absorptive capabilities and should not be used on infected wounds because bacteria and fungus can proliferate under this type of dressing.

Intravenous Extravasation

Clinical Practice	Referenced Rationale and Quality of Evidence Rating
Definition: *Intravenous extravasation* (formerly called infiltration) is the inadvertent leaking/administration of an infusing vesicant or nonvesicant solution or medication into the surrounding tissue instead of into the intended vascular pathway.	Neonates, especially those less than 26 weeks of gestation, are at high risk of developing extravasation injuries because of their immature skin structures, lack of subcutaneous tissue, and the small size of their blood vessels (**Amjad, Murphy, Nylander-Housholder, & Ranft, 2011: III; Sardesai et al., 2011: III**). While adverse outcomes from an infiltration can occur with even the most prudent care, prevention of adverse outcomes is optimal (**Doellman et al., 2009: III**). These injuries, including cosmetic and functional complications, and consequently, the surgical interventions required, may prolong hospitalization and have been associated with significant morbidity (**Amjad et al., 2011: III; Casanova, Bardot, & Magalon, 2001: II-3**). Many extravasations resulting in significant damage in newborns have been associated with the use of hypertonic solutions, use of infusion pumps, and prolonged administration of IV solutions with intermittent administration of medication (**Thigpen, 2007: III**). Early treatment is recommended to minimize duration of exposure and avoid skin necrosis at the site of infusion. Accumulating fluid exerts a mechanical pressure on the subdermal vessels, creating potential ischemic injuries. Compression of surrounding tissues by a large volume of infiltrate can result in an acute limb compartment syndrome (**Doellman et al., 2009: III**). If the infiltrate is from a vesicant fluid, additional damage to the subcutaneous tissue could occur because cells are basically "burned" by the vesicant infusion and begin to die. This severe consequence can progress unnoticed for 48–72 hours after infiltration (**Amjad et al., 2011: III**).
The following interventions are recommended to minimize the risk of extravasation: a. Use vascular access devices made of plastic materials instead of steel needles.	 Insertion devices covered with silicone catheters cause less damage to the vessel, last longer, are easier to stabilize, and carry less risk for infiltration than steel needles. A common catheter size for neonates is 24 gauge (**Frey & Pettit, 2010: III; Thigpen, 2007: III**). In infants, the average dwell time of infusion devices ranges from 15 hours for a steel needle to 54 hours for a catheter-style device (**Pettit, 2003: III**). Tissue damage from extravasation may cause disfigurement, functional limitations (**Gopalakrishnan, Goel, & Banerjee, 2012: III**), or, in rare cases, the loss of the extremity if vascular flow is obstructed.
b. Avoid placing vascular access devices in areas difficult to immobilize whenever possible, especially those near areas of flexion; surrounding tendons, nerves, or arteries;	Evaluate extremity immobilization for possible nerve compression, contracture formation, and pressure sores (**Pettit, 2003: III**). The choice of insertion site strongly influences the duration of peripheral IV therapy and the reason for catheter removal; when possible, initial IV sites should be inserted in the most distal part of the extremity (**Frey & Pettit, 2010: III; Sawatzky-Dicksson & Bodnaryk, 2006: II-3**).

Clinical Practice	Referenced Rationale and Quality of Evidence Rating
or near the face and forehead. • When choosing IV therapy sites, select veins in the most distal part of the extremity, whenever possible.	
c. Secure vascular access devices with transparent adhesive dressing.	Transparent adhesive dressings permit ongoing visualization of the insertion site and help to stabilize the catheter to prevent in-and-out movement of the catheter (**Lund & Kuller, 2007: III; Perucca, 2010: III**).
d. When using an arm board, prevent obstruction of venous return by placing tape loosely over bony prominences and do not completely encircle the extremity with tape.	Taping methods can constrict venous return, especially in extremities, and compromise blood flow (**Thigpen, 2007: III**).
e. Ideally, peripheral IV solutions that approximate physiologic osmolality as closely as possible should be administered.	Properties of an infusion solution or medication that influence risk of injury include its chemical properties, osmolality, and pH. Osmolality of a medication is a combination of the dose, the amount of solution prepared, and the type of diluents used (**Thigpen, 2007: III**). Normal serum osmolality is 280–295 mOsm/kg. To prevent damage to the peripheral vessel wall, IV solutions infused through a peripheral IV catheter should have an osmolality within this range. Hypertonic solutions may cause the cells to shrink by drawing fluid from them. Hypotonic solutions may cause cell rupture by drawing fluid into them (**Thigpen, 2007: III**).
f. Dextrose concentration administered peripherally should be limited to 10% to 12.5%, according to facility protocol.	Glucose concentrations that are greater than 12.5% administered through a peripheral IV can cause phlebitis and extravasation injury if an infiltration occurs. Higher concentrations of glucose may be delivered through central catheters (**Weinstein, 2007: III**). Chemical irritation of the inner lining of the blood vessel can results in thrombosis, inflammation, edema, or infiltration. Hypertonic or acidic electrolyte solutions may be especially deleterious when infiltrated (**Doellman et al., 2009: III**). Vasopressors, such as dopamine and epinephrine, produce intense local vasoconstriction and tissue ischemia (**Sardesai et al., 2011: III**).
g. Use recommended diluents prior to IV medication administration.	Medications that are diluted according to a standard reference (e.g., Lexicomp®, NeoFax® or another standard reference) help prevent precipitate formation that can result in occlusion and also help prevent irritation of the inner lining of the vessel (**Perucca, 2010: III**).

2

Clinical Practice	Referenced Rationale and Quality of Evidence Rating
Assess the catheter–skin junction site, surrounding tissue and the catheter tip site for swelling, redness, blanching, signs of pain, or leakage at least every hour or according to facility protocol. Document these signs and the integrity of the transparent dressing that covers the site. • Do not rely on infusion pumps to detect infiltration.	Hourly assessments can prevent or minimize the risk of infiltration. Observations should be more frequent during infusion of more irritating medications or solutions (**Sawatzky-Dicksson & Bodnaryk, 2006: II-3; Shah & Sinha, Ng, & Sinha, 2011: III; Simona, 2012: III**). Infusion pumps should not be counted on to detect infiltrations, as these devices will detect an infiltration only after fluid has already collected in the surrounding tissue (**Amjad et al., 2011: III; Infusion Nurses Society, 2011: III**).
a. If signs of extravasation are noted, stop the infusion immediately. Signs and symptoms of infiltration include swelling, pain at the site, blanching or coolness of the skin, inability to flush, leakage at the site, or erythema. In severe cases, there may be blister formation and subsequent tissue sloughing.	Checking for blood return is not an accurate method of determining catheter patency because the small catheter size may prevent the withdrawal of blood even when the catheter is patent (**Fabian, 2000: III; Pettit, 2003: III**). Also, there may be good blood return even with infiltration of solution. Edema and inflammation result in vasoconstriction that worsens the tissue damage.
b. Consider using an objective scale to determine degree of extravasation. Some examples include but are not limited to the following: • Milliam Scale of IV Infiltrations • Infusion Nurses Society Thigpen Grading Scale of IV Infiltrations • Revised Grading Scale of IV Infiltrations • Pediatric IV Infiltration Scale	The use of an infiltration scale for treatment of IV infiltrations may minimize adverse outcomes by improving communication and consistency of treatment (**Amjad et al., 2011: III; Sawatzky-Dicksson & Bodnaryk, 2006: II-3; Simona, 2012: III**). Assigning the degree of extravasation injury can aid in determining the appropriate treatment (**Thigpen, 2007: III**). Several infiltration grading scales have been developed. The Milliam Scale refers to the number of the joints involved rather than the number of inches involved, thus reflecting the degree of severity relative to the size of the patient and not the size of the infiltrate (**Amjad et al., 2011: III**). The Thigpen Grading Scale delineates the treatment options relative to the nurse's observation of the condition of extravasated tissue (**Thigpen, 2007: III**). Complete and accurate documentation of the infiltration event and interventions should be performed and is facilitated with the use of a comprehensive, standardized form (**Doellman et al., 2009: III**).

3 Implement one or more of the following treatment options for IV extravasation as indicated and according to facility protocol:

The goal of treatment is to improve tissue perfusion and prevent progressive tissue necrosis. Treatment decisions are based on size and appearance of the injury, type of IV fluid infused, duration of exposure, and location. Initial signs of visible damage do not necessarily reflect underlying tissue damage. Deeper sloughing and tissue necrosis may occur over days to weeks (**Thigpen, 2007: III**). There is currently no research data comparing outcomes of various treatment modalities. Therefore, treatment has not been standardized and usually varies among facilities. Specific therapies are based on the assessment of the degree of injury, with invasive methods reserved for severe stages of injury (**Sardesai et al., 2011: III**).

a. Nonpharmacologic interventions for IV extravasation may include but are not limited to the following:

- Elevate the site of an IV extravasation or the affected extremity.

Immediate elevation of the affected site will aid venous return, facilitate fluid reabsorption, and sometimes prevent serious complications (Casanova et al., 2001: II-3; Ramasethu, 2004: III; Doellman et al., 2009: III).

- Using aseptic technique, make multiple puncture holes over the area of greatest swelling and gently squeeze or let the extravasated fluid leak out of the tissue to remove the infiltrate and prevent skin sloughs.

The multiple puncture technique has been reported to dramatically improve the swelling within a few hours and result in complete recovery within 24 hours. The potential for infection and additional tissue trauma exists (**Chandavasu, Garrow, Valda, Alsjeikh, & Dela Vega, 1986: III; Sawatzky-Dicksson & Bodnaryk, 2006: II-3**). Use measures to improve comfort and alleviate pain as needed.

Techniques involving saline washout and liposuction or some combination of these steps have been reported. The goal of these techniques is to remove most of the toxic agent remaining in the tissues. The procedure is accomplished by making four small incisions around the periphery of the extravasation. Large volumes of saline are then infused into one incision and flow out from the other three incisions (**Casanova et al., 2001: II-3; Davies, Gault, & Buchdahl, 1994: III; Gault, 1993: III**).

b. Pharmacologic interventions for IV extravasation may include the following:

- Administer the appropriate therapeutic agent as soon as possible but no later than 12 hours after the infiltrate is identified.

Pharmacologic treatment tends to be most effective if it occurs within 1 hour of infiltration (**Laurie, Wilson, Kernahan, Bauer, & Vistnes, 1984: II-1; Ramasethu, 2004: III**) but may still be effective if administered within 12 hours (**Flemmer & Chan, 1993: III**). The longer the tissue is exposed to the extravasated solution, the greater the chance of tissue damage.

- Hyaluronidase may be used for many types of IV extravasation.
  - i. After disinfection, subcutaneously administer four to five 0.2-mL injections in a circular pattern around the peripheral edge of the infiltration.
  - ii. Do not administer medication through the IV catheter.

Hyaluronidase is a protein enzyme that causes a reduction in inflammation and a rapid diffusion of the extravasated fluids through tissue by temporarily dissolving normal interstitial barriers, thereby decreasing tissue damage from the toxic substance (**Beaulieu, 2012: III; Kuensting, 2011: III; Sawatzky-Dicksson & Bodnaryk, 2006: II-3**). Hyaluronidase acts rapidly, usually within 10 minutes, and results in diffusion of extravasated fluid over an area that is typically three to five times larger than an untreated area (**Doellman et al., 2009: III**).
In vitro studies suggest hyaluronidase may decrease the morbidity associated with IV extravasation injury. Hyaluronidase should not be administered through the IV catheter prior to removal because the enzyme is rapidly inactivated (**Beaulieu, 2012: III**).The needle should be changed

Clinical Practice	Referenced Rationale and Quality of Evidence Rating
iii. Change the needle with each injection.	between each subcutaneous injection to avoid bacterial contamination (**Beaulieu, 2012: III; Thigpen, 2007: III**).
• Phentolamine is the antidote for extravasation of alpha adrenergic agents that cause vasoconstriction, such as dopamine and norepinephrine. i. The recommended dose is 0.01 mg/kg per dose, up to 5 mL of a 1 mg/mL solution diluted to 1 mL. ii. Administer subcutaneously around the periphery of the extravasation in four to five 0.2-mL injections.	Phentolamine has been used when a vasoactive medication (such as dopamine) has infiltrated and the skin appears pale, cold, and firm (**Thigpen, 2007: III**). It should be given within 12 hours. A marked decrease in swelling may occur within 15–30 minutes after administration (**Buck, 1998: III**). The use of repeated small doses may be best, because hypotension is a potential complication (**Ramasethu, 2004: III**). Blood pressure may drop because of the vasodilatation effects of phentolamine and the precipitous discontinuation or disruption of the drug that infiltrated (**Thigpen, 2007: III**).
• Nitroglycerin 2% may be a safe and effective treatment of cutaneous skin or tissue ischemia. i. Monitor for signs of hypotension and tachycardia	Transdermal nitroglycerin patches containing 2.5 mg of glyceryl trinitrate or topical 2% nitroglycerin ointment are well absorbed across intact skin (**Denkler & Cohen, 1989: III**). Nitroglycerin should be used with caution in infants with skin breakdown because of the variable absorption rates (**Flemmer & Chan, 1993: III; Thigpen, 2007: III**). Close monitoring of vital signs is important to identify early side effects (**Varughese & Koh, 2001: III**).
4 Choose an occlusive dressing that provides: • exudate management, • adherence without damaging the surrounding tissue, • a microbial barrier, • debridement, and • compression.	The positive effects of moisture on wound healing include facilitation of epidermal regeneration, endothelial cell proliferation, fibroblast proliferation, and prevention of scarring (**Sawatzky-Dicksson & Bodnaryk, 2006: II-3; Taquino, 2000: III**). Therefore, choose a product that maintains an occlusive barrier for healing. Appropriate selection of a wound management product is important, because atraumatic dressing removal is essential to minimize further injury and reduce pain (**Fox, 2011: III**).
a. Hydrocolloid dressings	Occlusive hydrocolloid dressings provide a bacterial barrier and a lower pH that inhibits the growth of pathogens. The serous fluid that accumulates under these dressings contains a higher level of keratinocytes and functioning neutrophils than other dressing types, promoting rapid wound healing (**Irving, 1999: III; Sawatzky-Dicksson & Bodnaryk, 2006: II-3**).
b. Hydrogel sheets and amorphous gel	Hydrogels consist of 80–90% water, which is soothing and gentle to skin and keeps the wound moist (**Cisler-Cahill, 2006: II-3**). Hydrogels facilitate autodebridement of wounds by rehydrating sloughing tissue and enhancing the rate of autolysis. In laboratory studies, hydrogels have

	Clinical Practice	Referenced Rationale and Quality of Evidence Rating
		been shown to exert a mild bactericidal effect because of the propylene glycol that most contain. Two forms of hydrogels are currently available: amorphous gel and sheet dressings. The choice of product is based on the type and site of the wound, as well as the fluid-handling capacity needed (**Cisler-Cahill, 2006: II-3; Lehr et al., 2004: II-3**). Gel over the wound enclosed in a polythene bag, forming a glove or boot, has been used to treat wounds caused by IV infiltrates (**Thomas et al., 1997: II-3**). It is also possible to combine the effects of hydrogel and hydrocolloid by applying hydrogel and covering it with hydrocolloid dressing.
5	For an extensive extravasation, consultation with a plastic surgeon or dermatologist may be considered.	Full-thickness injury carries the potential need for surgical debridement and skin grafting (**Thigpen, 2007: III**).
6	The following interventions are *discouraged* in most cases in the neonatal population because of the lack of research, potential for toxicity, or other detrimental effects, despite the fact that case reports that support use exist in the literature:	
	a. Topical application of silver sulfadiazine cream to the wound	Silver sulfadiazine cream is not recommended for neonates, because sulfur-containing medications compete with bilirubin for binding to albumin. Unbound bilirubin is then available for absorption through the blood–brain barrier and can potentially result in kernicterus. It is contraindicated in premature or newborn infants up to 2 months of age (**Bree & Siegfried, 2008: III**).
	b. Topical application of heat or cold	The effect of application of heat or cold to IV infiltration sites has not been studied in the neonatal population; no evidence supports or refutes the safety and efficacy of these practices. Considering the risk of thermal injury in already compromised, immature, and possibly hypoperfused skin, application of heat or cold is discouraged (**Doellman et al., 2009: III; Fabian, 2000: III; Ramasethu, 2004: III; Thigpen 2007: III**). The application of moist heat should be avoided because it can lead to tissue maceration and subsequent necrosis (**Banta & Noerr, 1992: III; Brown, Hoelzer, & Piercy, 1979: II-2**).

REFERENCES

Neonatal Skin Care

Abraham, G. (2007). Exogenous Cushing's syndrome induced by surreptitious topical glucocorticosteroid overdose in infants with diaper dermatitis. *Journal of Pediatric Endocrinology & Metabolism: JPEM, 20,* 1169–1171.

Adam, R., Schnetz, B., Mathey, P., Pericoi, M., & De Prost, Y. (2009). Clinical demonstration of skin mildness and suitability for sensitive infant skin of a new baby wipe. *Pediatric Dermatology, 26,* 506–513. doi:10.1111/j.1525-1470.2008.00804.x

Agren, J., Sjors, G., & Sedin, G. (1998). Transepidermal water loss in infants born at 24 and 25 weeks of gestation. *Acta Paediatrica, 87,* 1185–1190.

Agren J., Sjors G., & Sedin G. (2006). Ambient humidity influences the rate of skin barrier maturation in extremely preterm infants. *The Journal of Pediatrics, 148,* 613–617.

Ahmadpour-Kacho, M., Zahedpasha, Y., Hajian, K., Javadi, G., & Talebian, H. (2006). The effect of topical application of human milk, ethyl alcohol 96%, and silver sulfadiazine on umbilical cord separation time in newborn infants. *Archives of Iranian Medicine, 9,* 33–38.

Ahmed, A. S. M. N. U., Saha, S. K., Chowdhury, M. A. K. A., Law, P. A., Black, R. E., Santosham, M., & Darmstadt, G. L. (2007). Acceptability of massage with skin barrier-enhancing emollients in young neonates in Bangladesh. *Journal of Health, Population, and Nutrition, 25,* 236–240.

Akinbi, H., Narendran, V., Pass, A., Markart, P., & Hoath, S. (2004). Host defense proteins in vernix caseosa and amniotic fluid. *American Journal Obstetrics & Gynecology, 191,* 2090–2096.

Alberta, L., Sweeney, S. M., & Wiss, K. (2005). Diaper dye dermatitis. *Pediatrics, 116,* e450–e452. doi:10.1542/peds.2004-2066

Aly, R., Shirley, C., Cunico, B., & Maibach, H. I. (1978). Effect of prolonged occlusion on the microbial flora, pH, carbon dioxide and transepidermal water loss on human skin. *Journal of Investigative Dermatology, 71,* 378–381.

American Academy of Pediatrics. (2009). *Summer Safety Tips: Sun and Water Safety.* Retrieved from http://www.healthychildren.org/English/news/Pages/Summer-Safety-Tips-Sun-and-Water-Safety.aspx?nfstatus=401&nftoken=00000000-0000-0000-0000-000000000000&nfstatusdescription=ERROR%3a+No+local+token

American Academy of Pediatrics. (1999). Circumcision Policy Statement. *Pediatrics, 103,* 686–693.

American Academy of Pediatrics & American College of Obstetricians and Gynecologists. (2012). *Guidelines for perinatal care* (7th ed.). Elk Grove Village, IL: American Academy of Pediatrics; Washington, DC: American College of Obstetrics and Gynecology.

American Academy of Pediatrics & American Heart Association. (2010). *Neonatal resuscitation textbook* (6th ed.). Elk Grove Village, IL: American Academy of Pediatrics & American Heart Association.

Amjad, I., Murphy, T., Nylander-Housholder, L., & Ranft, A. (2011). A new approach to management of intravenous infiltration in pediatric patients: Pathophysiology, classification, and treatment. *Journal of Infusion Nursing, 34,* 242–249. doi:10.1097/NAN.0b013e31821da1b3

Ananthapadmanabhan, K. P., Moore, D. J., Subramanyan, K., Misra, M., & Meyer, F. (2004). Cleansing without compromise: the impact of cleansers on the skin barrier and the technology of mild cleansing. *Dermatologic Therapy, 17* (Suppl. 1), 16–25.

Andersen, C., Hart, J., Vemgal, P., & Harrison, C. (2005). Prospective evaluation of a multi-factorial prevention strategy on the impact of nosocomial infection in very-low-birthweight infants. *Journal of Hospital Infection, 61,* 162–167.

Anderson, G. C., Lane, A. E., & Chang, H. (1995). Axillary temperature in transitional newborn infants before and after tub bath. *Applied Nursing Research, 8,* 123–128.

Arifeen, S. E., Mullany, L. C., Shah, R., Mannan, I., Rahman, S. M., Talukder, M. R. R., … Baqui, A. H. (2012). The effect of cord cleansing with chlorhexidine on neonatal mortality in rural Bangladesh: A community-based, cluster-randomised trial. *Lancet, 379,* 1022–1028. doi:10.1016/S0140-6736(11)61848-5

Association of Women's Health, Obstetric and Neonatal Nurses. (2001) *Neonatal skin care: Evidence-based clinical practice guideline.* Washington, DC: Author.

Association of Women's Health, Obstetric and Neonatal Nurses. (2007). *Neonatal skin care: Evidence-based clinical practice guideline* (2nd ed.). Washington, DC: Author.

Association of Women's Health, Obstetric and Neonatal Nurses. (2010). *Assessment and care of the late preterm infant: Evidence-based clinical practice guideline.* Washington, DC: Author.

Atherton, D. (2005). Maintaining healthy skin in infancy using prevention of irritant napkin dermatitis as a model. *Community Practitioner: The Journal of the Community Practitioners' & Health Visitors' Association, 78,* 255–257.

Atherton, D. J. (2001). The aetiology and management of irritant diaper dermatitis. *Journal of the European Academy of Dermatology and Venereology, 15* (Suppl. 1), 1–4.

Atherton, D. J. (2004). A review of the pathophysiology, prevention and treatment of irritant diaper dermatitis. *Current Medical Research and Opinion, 20,* 645–649.

Aulbert, W., Parpart, C., Schulz-Hornbostel, R., Hinrichs, B., Krüger-Corcoran, D., & Stockfleth, E. (2009). Certification of sun protection practices in a German child day-care centre improves children's sun protection--the "SunPass" pilot study. *The British Journal of Dermatology, 161 Suppl 3,* 5–12. doi:10.1111/j.1365-2133.2009.09443.x

AvRuskin, T. W., Greenfield, E., Prasad, V., Greig, F., & Juan, C. S. (1994). Decreased T3 and T4 levels following topical application of povidone-iodine in premature neonates. *Journal of Pediatric Endocrinology, 7,* 205–209.

Baharestani, M. M. (2007). An overview of neonatal and pediatric wound care knowledge and considerations. *Ostomy Wound Management, 53,* 34–36.

Banta, C., & Noerr, B. (1992). Hyaluronidase. *Neonatal Network, 11,* 103–105.

Bautista, M. I., Wickett, R. R., Visscher, M. O., Pickens, W. L., Hoath, S. B. (2000). Characterization of vernix caseosa as a natural biofilm: Comparison to standard oil-based ointments. *Pediatric Dermatology, 17*, 253–260.

Beaulieu, M. J. (2012). Hyaluronidase for extravasation management. *Neonatal Network, 31*, 413–418. doi:10.1891/0730-0832.31.6.413

Beeram, M., Olvera, R., Krauss, D., Loughran, C., & Petty, M. (2006). Effects of topical emollient therapy on infants at or less than 27 weeks' gestation. *Journal of the National Medical Association, 98*, 261–264.

Behrendt, H., & Green, M. (1971). *Patterns of skin pH from birth through adolescence.* Springfield, IL: Charles C. Thomas.

Behring, A., Vezeau, T. M., & Fink, R. (2003). Timing of the newborn first bath: A replication. *Neonatal Network, 22*, 39–46.

Belghazi, K., Tourneux, P., Elabbassi, E. B., Ghyselen, L., Delanaud, S., & Libert, J. P. (2006). Effect of posture on the thermal efficiency of a plastic bag wrapping in neonate: Assessment using a thermal "sweating" mannequin. *Medical Physics, 33*, 637–644.

Benjamin, D. K., Jr., Stoll, B. J., Gantz, M. G., Walsh, M. C., Sánchez, P. J., Das, A., ... Goldberg, R. N. (2010). Neonatal candidiasis: Epidemiology, risk factors, and clinical judgment. *Pediatrics, 126*, e865–e873. doi:10.1542/peds.2009-3412

Berg, R. W. (1987). Etiologic factors in diaper dermatitis: A model for development of improved diapers. *Pediatrician, 14* (Suppl. 1), 27–33.

Berg, R. W., Buckingham, K. W., & Stewart, R. L. (1986). Etiologic factors in diaper dermatitis: The role of urine. *Pediatric Dermatology, 3*, 102–106.

Bertini, G., Perugi, S., Elia, S., Pratesi, S., Dani, C., & Rubaltelli, F. F. (2008). Transepidermal water loss and cerebral hemodynamics in preterm infants: Conventional versus LED phototherapy. *European Journal of Pediatrics, 167*, 37–42. doi:10.1007/s00431-007-0421-3

Bhatia, J. (2006). Fluid and electrolyte management in the very low birth weight neonate. *Journal of Perinatology, 26* (Suppl. 1), S19–S21. doi:10.1038/sj.jp.7211466

Bhandari, V., Brodsky, N., & Porat, R. (2005). Improved outcome of extremely low birth weight infants with Tegaderm application to skin. *Journal of Perinatology, 25*, 276–281.

Bieber, T. (2010). Atopic dermatitis. *Annals of Dermatology, 22*, 125–137. doi:10.5021/ad.2010.22.2.125

Bishay, M., Retrosi, G., Horn, V., Cloutman-Green, E., Harris, K., De Coppi, P., ... Pierro, A. (2011). Chlorhexidine antisepsis significantly reduces the incidence of sepsis and septicemia during parenteral nutrition in surgical infants. *Journal of Pediatric Surgery, 46*, 1064–1069. doi:10.1016/j.jpedsurg.2011.03.028

Bissinger, R. L., & Annibale, D. J. (2010). Thermoregulation in very low-birth-weight infants during the golden hour: Results and implications. *Advances in Neonatal Care, 10*, 230–238. doi:10.1097/ANC.0b013e3181f0ae63

Black, P. (2007). Peristomal skin care: An overview of available products. *British Journal of Nursing, 16*, 1048, 1050, 1052–1054, passim.

Blume-Peytavi, U., Cork, M. J., Faergemann, J., Szczapa, J., Vanaclocha, F., & Gelmetti, C. (2009). Bathing and cleansing in newborns from day 1 to first year of life: Recommendations from a European round table meeting. *Journal of the European Academy of Dermatology and Venereology, 23*, 751–759. doi:10.1111/j.1468-3083.2009.03140.x

Bolton, L. (2004). Moist wound healing from past to present. In D. T. Rovee & H. I. Maibach (Eds.), *Epidermis in wound healing* (pp. 89–102). Aberdeen, UK: CRC Press.

Brandon, D. H., Coe, K., Hudson-Barr, D., Oliver, T., & Landerman, L. R. (2010). Effectiveness of No-Sting skin protectant and Aquaphor on water loss and skin integrity in premature infants. *Journal of Perinatology, 30*, 414–419. doi:10.1038/jp.2009.174

Bree, A., & Siegfried, E. (2008). Neonatal skin care and toxicology. In L. F. Eichenfield, I. J. Frieden, & N. B. Esterly (Eds.), *Neonatal Dermatology* (2nd ed., pp. 59–72). Philadelphia: Saunders Elsevier.

Breternitz, M., Flach, M., Prässler, J., Elsner, P., & Fluhr, J. W. (2007). Acute barrier disruption by adhesive tapes is influenced by pressure, time and anatomical location: Integrity and cohesion assessed by sequential tape stripping. A randomized, controlled study. *British Journal of Dermatology, 156*, 231–240. doi:10.1111/j.1365-2133.2006.07632.x

Bridges, B. (2002). Fragrance: emerging health and environmental concerns. *Flavour and Fragrance Journal, 17*, 361-371. doi: 10.1002/ffj.1106

Bringué Espuny, X., Soria, X., Solé, E., Garcia, J., Marco, J. J., Ortega, J., ... Pueyo, A. (2010). Chlorhexidine-methanol burns in two extreme preterm newborns. *Pediatric Dermatology, 27*, 676–678.

Brook, I. (2002). Cutaneous and subcutaneous infections in newborns due to anaerobic bacteria. *Journal of Perinatal Medicine, 30*, 197–208.

Brown, A., Hoelzer, D., & Piercy, S. (1979). Skin necrosis from extravasation of intravenous fluids in children. *Plastic & Reconstructive Surgery, 64*, 145–150.

Brown-Trask, B., Van Sell, S., Carter, S., & Kindred, C. (2009). Circumcision care. *RN, 72*, 22–28.

Bryanton, J., Walsh, D., Barrett, M., & Gaudet, D. (2004). Tub bathing versus traditional sponge bathing for the newborn. *Journal of Obstetric, Gynecologic, and Neonatal Nursing, 33*, 704–712.

Buck, M. L. (1998). Treatment of intravenous extravasations. *Pediatric Pharmacotherapy: A Monthly Newsletter for Health Care Professionals, 4*, 1–4. Retrieved from http://www.medicine.virginia.edu/clinical/departments/pediatrics/education/pharm-news/1995-2000/199801.pdf

Bustamante, S. A., & Steslow, J. (1989). Use of a transparent adhesive dressing in very low birthweight infants. *Journal of Perinatology, 9*, 165–169.

Campbell, J. R., Zaccaria, E., & Baker, C. J. (2000). Systemic candidiasis in extremely low birth weight infants receiving topical petrolatum ointment for care: A case-control study. *Pediatrics, 105*, 1041–1045.

Campbell, R. L., Seymour, J. L., Stone, L. C., & Milligan, M. C. (1987). Clinical studies with disposable diapers containing absorbent gelling materials: Evaluation on infant skin condition. *Journal of the American Academy of Dermatology, 17*, 978–987.

Capone, K., Dowd, S., Stamatas, G., & Nikolovski, J. (2011.) Diversity of the human skin microbiome early in life. *Journal of Investigative Dermatology, 131*, 2026–2032.

Carey, A. J., & Long, S. S. (2010). *Staphylococcus aureus*: A continuously evolving and formidable pathogen in the neonatal intensive care unit. *Clinics in Perinatology, 37*, 535–546.

Casanova, D., Bardot, J., & Magalon, G. (2001). Emergency treatment of accidental infusion leakage in the newborn: Report of 14 cases. *British Journal of Plastic Surgery, 54*, 396–399.

Centers for Disease Control and Prevention. (2006). Leads from the MMWR. Update: Universal precautions for prevention of transmission of human immunodeficiency virus, hepatitis B virus, and other bloodborne pathogens in health care settings. *Journal of the American Medical Association, 260*, 462–465.

Centers for Disease Control and Prevention. (2011). *2011 Guidelines for the prevention of intravascular catheter-related infections.* Retrieved from http://www.cdc.gov/hicpac/BSI/BSI-guidelines-2011.html

Centers for Disease Control and Prevention (2013). *Hand hygiene in health care settings.* Retrieved from http://www.cdc.gov/handhygiene/

Chaiyakunapruk, N., Veenstra, D. L., Lipsky, B. A., & Saint, S. (2002). Chlorhexidine compared with povidone-iodine solution for vascular catheter-site care: A meta-analysis. *Annals of Internal Medicine, 136*, 792–801.

Chamnanvanakij, S., Decharachakul, K., Rasamimaree, P., & Vanprapar, N. (2005). A randomized study of 3 umbilical cord care regimens at home in Thai neonates: Comparison of time to umbilical cord separation, parental satisfaction and bacterial colonization. *Journal of the Medical Association of Thailand, 88*, 967–972.

Chan, L. (2008) Atopic dermatitis in 2008. *Current Directions in Autoimmunity, 10*, 76–118.

Chandavasu, O., Garrow, E., Valda, V., Alsjeikh, S., & Dela Vega, S. (1986). A new method for the prevention of skin sloughs and necrosis secondary to intravenous infiltration. *American Journal of Perinatology, 3*, 4–5.

Chapman, A. K., Aucott, S. W., & Milstone, A. M. (2012). Safety of chlorhexidine gluconate used for skin antisepsis in the preterm infant. *Journal of Perinatology, 32*, 4–9. doi:10.1038/jp.2011.148

Choudhuri, J., McQueen, R., Inoue, S., & Gordon, R. C. (1990). Efficacy of skin sterilization for a venipuncture with the use of commercially available alcohol or iodine pads. *American Journal of Infection Control, 18*, 82–85.

Cisler-Cahill, L. (2006). Protocol for the use of amorphous hydrogel to support wound healing in neonatal patients: An adjunct to nursing skin care. *Neonatal Network, 25*, 267–273.

Cole, J. G., Brissette, N., J., & Lunardi, B. (1999). Tub Baths or Sponge Baths for Newborn Infants? *Mother Baby Journal, 4*, 39–43.

Concannon, P., Gisoldi, E., Phillips, S., & Grossman R. (2001). Diaper dermatitis: A therapeutic dilemma. Results of a double-blind placebo controlled trial of miconazole nitrate 0.25%. *Pediatric Dermatology 18*, 149–155.

Conner, J. M., Soll, R. F., & Edwards, W. H. (2003). Topical ointment for preventing infection in preterm infants. *Cochrane Database of Systematic Reviews,* Issue 4, Art. No. CD001150. doi:10.1002/14651858.CD001150.pub2

Cork, M., Robinson, D., Vasilopoulos, Y., Ferguson, A., Moustafa, M., MacGowan, A., … Tazi-Ahnini, R. (2006). New perspectives on epidermal barrier dysfunction in atopic dermatitis: Gene-environment interactions. *Journal of Allergy and Clinical Immunology, 118*, 3–21.

Curley, M. A. Q., Razmus, I. S., Roberts, K. E., & Wypij, D. (2003). Predicting pressure ulcer risk in pediatric patients. *Nursing Research, 52,* 22–33.

Cutting, K. F. (2008). Impact of adhesive surgical tape and wound dressings on the skin, with reference to skin stripping. *Journal of Wound Care, 17*, 157–158, 160–162.

Da Cunha, M. L., & Procianoy, R. S. (2005). Effect of bathing on skin flora of preterm newborns. *Journal of Perinatology, 25*, 375–379.

Da Cunha, M. L., Procianoy, R. S., Franceschini, D. T., De Oliveira, L. L., & Cunha, M. L. (2008). Effect of the first bath with chlorhexidine on skin colonization with *Staphylococcus aureus* in normal healthy term newborns. *Scandinavian Journal of Infectious Diseases, 40*, 615–620. doi:10.1080/00365540801932447

Dadlani, C., & Orlow, S. J. (2008). Planning for a brighter future: a review of sun protection and barriers to behavioral change in children and adolescents. *Dermatology Online Journal, 14*(9), 1.

Dani, C., Martelli, E., Reali, F. M., Bertini, G., Panin, G., & Rubaltelli, F. (2001). Fiberoptic and conventional phototherapy effects on the skin of premature infants. *Journal of Pediatrics, 138,* 438–440.

Darmstadt, G., Badrawi, N., Law, P. A., Ahmed, S., Bashir, M., Iskander, I., … Santosham, M. (2004). Topically applied sunflower seed oil prevents invasive bacterial infections in preterm infants in Egypt. *Pediatric Infectious Disease Journal, 23*, 719–725.

Darmstadt, G., & Dinulos, J. (2000). Neonatal skin care. *Pediatric Clinics of North America, 47,* 757–782.

Darmstadt, G., Dinulos, J., & Miller, Z. (2000). Congenital cutaneous candidiasis: Clinical presentation, pathogenesis, and management guidelines. *Pediatrics, 105*, 438–444.

Darmstadt, G., & Saha, S. (2002). Traditional practice of oil massage of neonates in Bangladesh. *Journal of Health, Population and Nutrition, 20*, 184–188.

Darmstadt, G. L., Hossain, M. M., Choi, Y., Shirin, M., Mullany, L. C., Islam, M., & Saha, S. K. (2007). Safety and effect of chlorhexidine skin cleansing on skin flora of neonates in Bangladesh. *Pediatric Infectious Disease Journal, 26*, 492–495. doi:10.1097/01.inf.0000261927.90189.88

Darmstadt, G. L., Saha, S. K., Ahmed, A. S. M. N. U., Ahmed, S., Chowdhury, M. A. K. A., Law, P. A., … Santosham, M. (2008). Effect of skin barrier therapy on neonatal mortality rates in preterm infants in Bangladesh: A randomized, controlled, clinical trial. *Pediatrics, 121*, 522–529. doi:10.1542/peds.2007-0213

Darmstadt, G. L., Saha, S. K., Ahmed, A. S. M. N. U., Choi, Y., Chowdhury, M. A. K. A., Islam, M., Ahmed, S. (2007). Effect of topical emollient treatment of preterm neonates in Bangladesh on invasion of pathogens into the bloodstream. *Pediatric Research, 61*(5 Pt. 1), 588–593. doi:10.1203/pdr.0b013e3180459f75

Darmstadt, G. L., Saha, S. K., Ahmed, A. S. M. N. U., Chowdhury, M. A. K. A., Law, P. A., Ahmed, S., … Santosham, M. (2005). Effect of topical treatment with skin barrier-enhancing emollients on nosocomial infections in preterm infants in Bangladesh: A randomised controlled trial. *Lancet, 365*, 1039–1045. doi:10.1016/S0140-6736(05)71140-5

Davis, J. A., Leyden, J. J., Grove, G. L., & Raynor, W. J. (1989). Comparison of disposable diapers with fluff absorbent and fluff plus absorbent polymers: Effects on skin hydration, skin pH, and diaper dermatitis. *Pediatric Dermatology, 6*, 102–108.

Davies, J., Gault, D., & Buchdahl, R. (1994). Preventing the scars of neonatal intensive care. *Archives of Disease in Childhood, Fetal and Neonatal Edition, 70*, F50–F51.

Davies, M. W., Dore A. J., & Perissinotto, K. L. (2006). Topical vitamin A, or its derivatives, for treating and preventing napkin dermatitis in infants (Review). *Cochrane Database of Systematic Reviews*, Issue 4, Art. No.: CD004300. doi:10.1002/1451858.CD004300.pub2.

De Carvalho, M., Torrao, C. T., & Moreira, M. E. L. (2011). Mist and water condensation inside incubators reduce the efficacy of phototherapy. *Archives of Disease in Childhood, Fetal and Neonatal Edition*, *96*, F138–F140. doi:10.1136/adc.2010.189423

Denkler, K. & Cohen, B. (1989). Reversal of dopamine extravasation injury with topical nitroglycerin ointment, 1989. *Journal of Plastic and Reconstructive Surgery, 84,* 811-813.

Devlin, R. (2006). Invasive fungal infections caused by *Candida* and *Malassezia* species in the neonatal intensive care unit. *Advances in Neonatal Care, 6*, 68–77.

de Wet, P. M., Rode, H., van Dyk, A., & Millar, A. J. (1999). Perianal candidiosis: A comparative study with mupirocin and nystatin. *International Journal of Dermatology, 38*, 618–622.

Dinulos J. G. H., & Pace, N. C. (2008). Bacterial infections. In L. F. Eichenfield, I. J. Frieden, & N. B. Esterly (Eds.), *Textbook of neonatal dermatology* (2nd ed., pp. 173–191). Philadelphia: W. B. Saunders Co.

Ditzenberger, G. R. (2010). Nutritional management. In M. T. Verklan & M. Walden (Eds.), *Core curriculum for neonatal intensive care nursing* (4th ed., pp. 182–207). St. Louis, MO: Saunders Elsevier.

Dizon, M. V., Galzote, C., Estanislao, R., Mathew, N., & Sarkar, R. (2010). Tolerance of baby cleansers in infants: A randomized controlled trial. *Indian Pediatrics, 47*, 959–963.

Doellman, D., Hadaway, L., Bowe-Geddes, L. A., Franklin, M., LeDonne, J., Papke-O'Donnell, L., … Stranz, M. (2009). Infiltration and extravasation: Update on prevention and management. *Journal of Infusion Nursing, 32*, 203–211. doi:10.1097/NAN.0b013e3181aac042

Dominguez-Bello, M., Costello, E., Contreras, M., Magris, M., Hidalgo, G., Fierer, N., & Knight, R. (2010). Delivery mode shapes the acquisition and structure of the initial microbiota across multiple body habitats in newborns. *Proceedings of the National Academy of Sciences of the Unites States of America, 26*, 11971–11975.

Donahue, M. L., Phelps, D. L., Richter, S. E., & Davis, J. M. (1996). A semipermeable skin dressing for extremely low birth weight infants. *Journal of Perinatology, 16*, 20–26.

Donlon, C. R., & Furdon, S. A. (2002). Assessment of the umbilical cord outside of the delivery room. Part 2. *Advances in Neonatal Care, 2*, 187–197.

Dore, S., Buchan, D., Coulas, S., Hamber, L., Stewart, M., Cowan, D., & Jamieson, L. (1998). Alcohol versus natural drying for newborn cord care. *Journal of Obstetric, Gynecologic, and Neonatal Nursing, 27*, 621–627.

Drucker, D., & Marshall, N. (1995). Humidification without risk of infection in the Drager incubator 8000. *Neonatal Intensive Care, 8*, 44–46.

Dykes, P. J. (2007). The effect of adhesive dressing edges on cutaneous irritancy and skin barrier function. *Journal of Wound Care, 16*, 97–100.

Dykes, P. J., & Heggie, R. (2003). The link between the peel force of adhesive dressings and subjective discomfort in volunteer subjects. *Journal of Wound Care, 12*, 260–262.

Dykes, P. J., Heggie, R., & Hill, S. A. (2001). Effects of adhesive dressings on the stratum corneum of the skin. *Journal of Wound Care, 10*, 7–10.

Edwards, W., Conner, J., & Soll, R. (2004). The effect of prophylactic ointment therapy on nosocomial sepsis rates and skin integrity in infants with birth weights of 501–1000 g. *Pediatrics, 113*, 1195–1203.

Engle, W, Tomashek, K. M., Wallman, C., & Committee on Fetus and Newborn, American Academy of Pediatrics. (2007). "Late-Preterm" infants: A population at risk. *Pediatrics, 120*, 1390–1401.

Erasala, G. N., Romain, C., & Merlay, I. (2011). Diaper area and disposable diapers. *Current Problems in Dermatology, 40*, 83–89. doi:10.1159/000321057

Ertel, K. D. (2003). Bathing the term newborn: Personal cleanser considerations. In S. B. Hoath & H. I. Maibach (Eds.), *Neonatal skin: structure and function* (2nd ed., pp. 211–236), New York: Marcel Dekker, Inc.

Etienne, K. A., Subudhi, C. P. K., Chadwick, P. R., Settle, P., Moise, J., Magill, S. S., … Balajee, S. A. (2011). Investigation of a cluster of cutaneous aspergillosis in a neonatal intensive care unit. *Journal of Hospital Infection, 79*, 344–348. doi:10.1016/j.jhin.2011.06.012

Evens, K., George, J., Angst, D., & Schweig, L. (2004). Does umbilical cord care in preterm infants influence cord bacterial colonization or detachment? *Journal of Perinatology, 24*, 100–104.

Fabian, B. (2000). Intravenous complication: Infiltration. *Journal of IV Nursing, 23*, 229–231.

Farrington, E. (1992). Diaper dermatitis. *Pediatric Nursing, 18*, 81–82.

Fern, D., Graves, C., & L'Huillier, M. (2002). Swaddled bathing in the newborn intensive care unit. *Newborn and Infant Nursing Reviews, 2*, 3–4. doi:10.1053/nbin.2002.31481

Fields, K. S., Nelson, T., & Powell, D. (2006). Contact dermatitis caused by baby wipes. Case letter. *Journal of the American Academy of Dermatology, 54*, s230–s232.

Fischer, C., Bertelle, V., Hohlfeld, J., Forcada-Guex, M., Stadelmann-Diaw, C., & Tolsa, J.-F. (2010). Nasal trauma due to continuous positive airway pressure in neonates. *Archives of Disease in Childhood, Fetal and Neonatal Edition, 95*, F447–F451. doi:10.1136/adc.2009.179416

Flemmer, L., & Chan, J. (1993). A pediatric protocol for management of extravasation injuries. *Pediatric Nursing, 19*, 355–358.

Fluhr, J. W., Darlenski, R., Taieb, A., Hachem, J.-P., Baudouin, C., Msika, P., … Berardesca, E. (2010). Functional skin adaptation in infancy — almost complete but not fully competent. *Experimental Dermatology, 19*, 483–492. doi:10.1111/j.1600-0625.2009.01023.x

Fortunov, R., Hulten, K., Hammerman, W., Mason, E., & Kaplan, S. (2006). Community-acquired *Staphylococcus aureus* infections in term and near-term previously healthy neonates. *Pediatrics, 118*, 874–882.

Fox, C., Nelson, D., & Wareham, J. (1998). The timing of skin acidification in very low birth weight infants. *Journal of Perinatology, 18*, 272–275.

Fox, M. D. (2011). Wound care in the neonatal intensive care unit. *Neonatal Network, 30*, 291–303. doi:10.1891/0730-0832.30.5.291

Frey, A., & Pettit, J. (2010). Infusion therapy in children. In M. Alexander, A. Corrigan, L. Gorski, J. Hankins, & R. Perucca (Eds.), *Infusion nursing: An evidence-based approach* (3rd ed., pp. 550–570). St. Louis, MO: Saunders Elsevier.

Fujii, K., Sugama, J., Okuwa, M., Sanada, H., & Mizokami, Y. (2010). Incidence and risk factors of pressure ulcers in seven neonatal intensive care units in Japan: a multisite prospective cohort study. *International Wound Journal, 7*, 323–328. doi:10.1111/j.1742-481X.2010.00688.x

Garcia Bartels, N., Mleczko, A., Schink, T., Proquitté, H., Wauer, R. R., & Blume-Peytavi, U. (2009). Influence of bathing or washing on skin barrier function in newborns during the first four weeks of life. *Skin Pharmacology and Physiology, 22*, 248–257. doi:10.1159/000235552

Garcia Bartels, N., Scheufele, R., Prosch, F., Schink, T., Proquitté, H., Wauer, R. R., & Blume-Peytavi, U. (2010). Effect of standardized skin care regimens on neonatal skin barrier function in different body areas. *Pediatric Dermatology, 27*, 1–8. doi:10.1111/j.1525-1470.2009.01068.x

Garland, J. S., Alex, C. P., Mueller, C. D., Otten, D., Shivpuri, C., Harris M. C., … Maki, D. G. (2001). A randomized trial comparing povidone-iodine to chlorhexidine gluconate-impregnated dressing for prevention of central venous catheter infections in neonates. *Pediatrics, 107*, 1431–1436.

Garland, J. S., Alex, C. P., Uhing, M. R., Peterside, I. E., Rentz, A., & Harris, M. C. (2009). Pilot trial to compare tolerance of chlorhexidine gluconate to povidone-iodine antisepsis for central venous catheter placement in neonates. *Journal of Perinatology, 29*, 808–813. doi:10.1038/jp.2009.161

Garland, J. S., Buck, R. K., Maloney, P., Durkin, D. M., Toth-Lloyd, S., Duffy, M., … Goldmann, D. (1995). Comparison of 10% povidone-iodine and 0.5% chlorhexidine gluconate for the prevention of peripheral intravenous catheter colonization in neonates: A prospective trial. *Pediatric Infectious Disease Journal, 14*, 510–516.

Gault, D. (1993). Extravasation injuries. *British Journal of Plastic Surgery, 46*, 91–96.

Gaylord, M., Wright, K., Lorch, K., Lorch, V., & Walker, E. (2001). Improved fluid management utilizing humidified incubators in extremely low birth weight infants. *Journal of Perinatology, 21*, 438–443.

Gelbaum, I. (1993). Circumcision: Refining a traditional surgical technique. *Journal of Nurse-Midwifery, 38,* 18S–30S.

Gfatter, R., Hackl P., & Braun, F. (1997). Effects of soap and detergents on skin surface pH, stratum corneum hydration and fat content in infants. *Dermatology, 195,* 258–262.

Ghadially, R., Halkier-Sorensen, L., & Elias, P. M. (1992). Effects of petrolatum on stratum corneum structure and function. *Journal of the American Academy of Dermatology, 26,* 387–396.

Gill, N. (1982). Benzoin contains many acids [Letter to the Editor]. *American Journal of Nursing, 82,* 244.

Golombek, S. G., Brill, P. E., & Salice, A. L. (2002). Randomized trial of alcohol versus triple dye for umbilical cord care. *Clinical Pediatrics, 41,* 419–423.

Gopalakrishnan, P., Goel, N., & Banerjee, S. (2012). Saline irrigation for the management of skin extravasation injury in neonates. *Cochrane Database of Systematic Reviews*, Issue 2, Art. No. 3: CD008404. doi:10.1002/14651858.CD008404

Gordon, C., Rowitch, D., Mitchell, M., & Kohane, I. (1995). Topical iodine and neonatal hypothyroidism. *Archives of Pediatrics and Adolescent Medicine, 149,* 1336–1339.

Gordon, M., & Montgomery, L. A. (1996). Minimizing epidermal stripping in the very low birth weight infant: Integrating research and practice to affect infant outcome. *Neonatal Network, 15,* 37–44.

Gotschall, C. S., Morrison, M., & Eichelberger, M. (1998). Prospective, randomized study of the efficacy of Mepitel on children with partial-thickness scalds. *Journal of Burn Care and Rehabilitation, 19,* 279–283.

Goujon, E., Beer, F., Gay, S., Sandre, D., Gouyon, J.-B., & Vabres, P. (2010). Anetoderma of prematurity: An iatrogenic consequence of neonatal intensive care. *Archives of Dermatology, 146,* 565–567. doi:10.1001/archdermatol.2010.65

Gregory, K. (2011). Microbiome aspects of perinatal and neonatal health. *Journal of Perinatal and Neonatal Nursing, 25,* 158–162.

Grunhagen, D. J., De Boer, M. G. J., De Beaufort, A. J., & Walther, F., (2001). Transepidermal water loss during halogen spotlight phototherapy in preterm infants. *Pediatrics Research, 51,* 402–405.

Guala, A., Pastore, G., Garipoli, V., Agosti, M., Vitali, M., & Bona, G. (2003). The time of umbilical cord separation in healthy full-term newborns: A controlled clinical trial of different cord care practices. *European Journal of Pediatrics, 162,* 350–351.

Hammarlund, K., & Sedin, G. (1979). Transepidermal water loss in newborn infants. III. Relation to gestational age. *Acta Paediatrica Scandinavica, 68,* 795–801.

Harpin, V., & Rutter, N. (1982). Percutaneous alcohol absorption and skin necrosis in a preterm infant. *Archives of Disease in Childhood, 57,* 477–479.

Harpin, V. A., & Rutter, N. (1983). Barrier properties of the newborn infant's skin. *Journal of Pediatrics, 102,* 419–425.

Harpin, V. A., & Rutter, N. (1985). Humidification of incubators. *Archives of Disease in Childhood, 60,* 219–224.

Harris, A. H., Coker, K. L., Smith, C. G., Uitvlugt, N., & Doctor, B. (2003). Case report of a pressure ulcer in an infant receiving extracorporeal life support: The use of a novel mattress surface for pressure reduction. *Advances in Neonatal Care, 3,* 220–229.

Haubrich, K. (2003). Role of vernix caseosa in the neonate: Potential application in the adult population. *AACN Clinical Issues, 14,* 457–464.

Heath, C., Desai, N., & Silverberg, N. B. (2009). Recent microbiological shifts in perianal bacterial dermatitis: *Staphylococcus aureus* predominance. *Pediatric Dermatology, 26,* 696–700. doi:10.1111/j.1525-1470.2009.01015.x

Heimall, L. M., Storey, B., Stellar, J. J., & Davis, K. F. (2012). Beginning at the bottom: Evidence-based care of diaper dermatitis. *MCN: The American Journal of Maternal Child Nursing, 37,* 10–16. doi:10.1097/NMC.0b013e31823850ea

Hennigsson, A., Nystrom, B., & Tunnel, R. (1981). Bathing or washing babies after birth. *Lancet, 19,* 1401–1403.

Hoath, S. & Pickens, W.L. (2003). Biology of vernix. In S. B. Hoath & H. I. Maibach (Eds.), *Neonatal skin: structure and function* (2nd ed., pp. 175-193). New York: Marcel Dekker, Inc.

Hoath, S., Narendran, V., & Visscher, M. O. (2001). The biology and role of vernix. *Newborn and Infant Nursing Reviews, 1,* 53–58.

Hodgins, S., Thapa, K., Khanal, L., Aryal, S., Suvedi, B. K., Baidya, U., & Mullany, L. C. (2010). Chlorhexidine gel versus aqueous for preventive use on umbilical stump: A randomized noninferiority trial. *Pediatric Infectious Disease Journal, 29,* 999–1003. doi:10.1097/INF.0b013e3181e70c59

Hoeger, P. H., Stark, S., & Jost, G. (2010). Efficacy and safety of two different antifungal pastes in infants with diaper dermatitis: A randomized, controlled study. *Journal of the European Academy of Dermatology and Venereology, 24,* 1094–1098. doi:10.1111/j.1468-3083.2010.03735.x

Holbrook, K. A. (1982). A histological comparison of infant and adult skin. In H. I. Maibach & E. K. Boisits (Eds.), *Neonatal skin: Structure and function* (1st ed., pp. 3–31). New York: Marcel Dekker, Inc.

Hook, K. P., & Eichenfield, L. F. (2011). Approach to the neonate with ecchymoses and crusts. *Dermatologic Therapy, 24,* 240–248. doi:10.1111/j.1529-8019.2011.01399.x

Hopkins, J. (2004). Essentials of newborn skin care. *British Journal of Midwifery, 12*: 314–317.

Hsu, W.-C., Yeh, L.-C., Chuang, M.-Y., Lo, W.-T., Cheng, S.-N., & Huang, C.-F. (2010). Umbilical separation time delayed by alcohol application. *Annals of Tropical Paediatrics, 30,* 219–223. doi:10.1179/14653281 0X12786388978643

Huffines B., & Logsdon, M. C. (1997). The neonatal skin risk assessment scale for predicting skin breakdown in neonates. *Issues in Comprehensive Pediatric Nursing, 20,* 103–114.

Humphrey, S., Bergman, J. N., & Au, S. (2006). Practical management strategies for diaper dermatitis. *Skin Therapy Letter, 11,* 1–6.

Irving, V. (1999). Neonatal iatrogenic skin injuries: A nursing perspective. *Journal of Neonatal Nursing, 5*, 10–14.

Irving, V. (2001). Reducing the risk of epidermal stripping in the neonatal population: An evaluation of an alcohol free barrier film. *Journal of Neonatal Nursing, 7*, 5–8.

Ittman, P. I., & Bozynski, M. E. (1993). Toxic epidermal necrolysis in a newborn infant after exposure to adhesive remover. *Journal of Perinatology, 13*, 476–477.

Jackson, P. D. (2010). Diaper dermatitis. Protecting the bottom line. *Advance for Nurse Practitioners, 18*, 35–36, 38–41.

Janssen, P. A., Selwood, B. L., Dobson, S. R., Peacock, D., & Thiessen, P. N. (2003). To dye or not to dye? A randomized, clinical trial of a triple dye/alcohol regime versus dry cord care. *Pediatrics, 111*, 15–20.

Jarrar, R., Buchhalter, J., Williams, K., McKay, M., & Luketich, C. (2011). Technical tips: Electrode safety in pediatric prolonged EEG recordings. *American Journal of Electroneurodiagnostic Technology, 51*, 114–117.

Johnson, C., & Versalovic, J. (2012). The human microbiome and its potential importance to pediatrics. *Pediatrics, 129*, 950–960.

Jones, S. (2000). Neonatal wound dehiscence and the subsequent healing process: A case study. *Ostomy Wound Management, 46*, 42–45, 48–50.

Kalia, Y. N., Nonato, L. B., Lund, C. H., & Guy, R. H. (1998). Development of skin barrier function in premature infants. *Journal of Investigative Dermatology, 111*, 320–326.

Kaufman, D. (2003). Strategies for prevention of neonatal invasive candidiasis. *Seminars in Perinatology, 27*, 414–424.

Kaufman, M. W., Clark, J., & Castro, C. (2001). Neonatal circumcision: Benefits, risks, and family teaching. *MCN: The American Journal of Maternal Child Nursing, 26*, 197–201.

Kayed, N. S., Farstad, H., & van der Meer, A. L. H. (2008). Preterm infants' timing strategies to optical collisions. *Early human development, 84*, 381–388. doi:10.1016/j.earlhumdev.2007.10.006

Khashu, M., Chessex, P., & Chanoine, J.-P. (2005). Iodine overload and severe hypothyroidism in a premature neonate. *Journal of Pediatric Surgery, 40*, E1–E4. doi:10.1016/j.jpedsurg.2004.10.028

Kiechl-Kohlendorfer, U., Berger, C., & Inzinger, R. (2008). The effect of daily treatment with an olive oil/lanolin emollient on skin integrity in preterm infants: A randomized controlled trial. *Pediatric Dermatology, 25*, 174–178. doi:10.1111/j.1525-1470.2008.00627.x

Kim, S. M., Lee, E. Y., Chen, J., & Ringer, S. A. (2010). Improved care and growth outcomes by using hybrid humidified incubators in very preterm infants. *Pediatrics, 125*, e137–e145. doi:10.1542/peds.2008-2997

Kjartansson, S., Arsan, S., Hammarlund, K., Sjors, G., & Sedin, G. (1995). Water loss from the skin of term and preterm infants nursed under a radiant heater. *Pediatrics Research, 37*, 233–238.

Kjartansson, S., Hammarlund, K., & Sedin, G. (1992). Insensible water loss from the skin during phototherapy in term and preterm infants. *Acta Paediatrica, 81*, 764–768.

Knauth, A., Gordin, M., McNelis, W., & Baumgart, S. (1989). Semipermeable polyurethane membrane as an artificial skin for the premature neonate. *Pediatrics, 83*, 945–950.

Knight, B. A., Puy, R., Douglass, J., O'Hehir, R. E., & Thien, F. (2001). Chlorhexidine anaphylaxis: A case report and review of the literature. *Internal Medicine Journal, 31*, 436–437.

Knobel, R. B., Simmer, J. E., & Holbert, D. (2005). Heat loss prevention for preterm infants in the delivery room. *Journal of Perinatology, 25*, 304–308.

Korting, H. C., & Braun-Falco, O. (1996). The effect of detergents on skin pH and its consequences. *Clinics in dermatology, 14*(1), 23–27.

Kosemund, K., Schlatter, H., Ochsenhirt, J. L., Krause, E. L., Marsman, D. S., & Erasala, G. N. (2009). Safety evaluation of superabsorbent baby diapers. *Regulatory Toxicology and Pharmacology, 53*, 81–89. doi:10.1016/j.yrtph.2008.10.005

Kuehl, B. L., Fyfe, K. S., & Shear, N. H. (2003). Cutaneous cleansers. *Skin Therapy Letter, 8*(3), 1–4.

Kuensting, L. L. (2010). Treatment of intravenous infiltration in a neonate. *Journal of Pediatric Health Care, 24*, 184–188. doi:10.1016/j.pedhc.2010.02.001

Kugelman, A., Inbar-Sanado, E., Shinwell, E. S., Makhoul, I. R., Leshem, M., Zangen, S., ... Bader, D. (2008). Iatrogenesis in neonatal intensive care units: Observational and interventional, prospective, multicenter study. *Pediatrics, 122*, 550–555. doi:10.1542/peds.2007-2729

Lane, A. T., & Drost, S. S. (1993). Effects of repeated application of emollient cream to premature neonates' skin. *Pediatrics, 92*, 415–419.

Laroia, N., Phelps, D. L., & Roy, J. (2007). Double wall versus single wall incubator for reducing heat loss in very low birth weight infants in incubators. *Cochrane Database of Systematic Reviews*, Issue 2, Art No.: CD004215. doi:10.1002/14651858.CD004215.pub2

Larson, A., & Dinulos, J. (2005). Cutaneous bacterial infections in the newborn. *Current Opinions in Pediatrics, 17*, 480.

Lashkari, H. P., Chow, P., & Godambe, S. (2012). Aqueous 2% chlorhexidine-induced chemical burns in an extremely premature infant. *Archives of Disease in Childhood, Fetal and Neonatal Edition, 97*, F64. doi:10.1136/adc.2011.215145

Laurie, S., Wilson, K., Kernahan, D., Bauer, B., & Vistnes, L. (1984). Intravenous extravasation injuries: The effectiveness of hyaluronidase in their treatment. *Annals of Plastic Surgery, 13*, 191–194.

Lavender, T., Furber, C., Campbell, M., Victor, S., Roberts, I., Bedwell, C., & Cork, M. J. (2012). Effect on skin hydration of using baby wipes to clean the napkin area of newborn babies: Assessor-blinded randomised controlled equivalence trial. *BMC Pediatrics, 12*, 59. doi:10.1186/1471-2431-12-59

LeBlanc, M. H. (1991). Thermoregulation: Incubators, radiant warmers, artificial skins, and body hoods. *Clinics in Perinatology, 18*, 403–422.

Lee, A., Harlan, R., Breaud, A. R., Speck, K., Perl, T. M., Clarke, W., & Milstone, A. M. (2011). Blood concentrations of chlorhexidine in hospitalized children undergoing daily chlorhexidine bathing. *Infection Control and Hospital Epidemiology, 32*, 395–397. doi:10.1086/659154

LeFevre, A., Shillcutt, S. D., Saha, S. K., Ahmed, A. S. M. N. U., Ahmed, S., Chowdhury, M. A., ... Darmstadt, G. L. (2010). Cost-effectiveness of skin-barrier-enhancing emollients among preterm infants in Bangladesh. *Bulletin of the World Health Organization, 88*, 104–112. doi:10.2471/BLT.08.058230

Ligi, I., Arnaud, F., Jouve, E., Tardieu, S., Sambuc, R., & Simeoni, U. (2008). Iatrogenic events in admitted neonates: A prospective cohort study. *Lancet, 371*(9610), 404–410. doi:10.1016/S0140-6736(08)60204-4

Liaw, J.-J., Yang, L., Yuh, Y.-S., & Yin, T. (2006). Effects of tub bathing procedures on preterm infants' behavior. *Journal of Nursing Research, 14*, 297–305.

Lehr, V., Luli-Butica, M., Lindblad, W., Kazzi, N., & Aranda, J. (2004). Management of the infiltration injury in neonates using DuoDerm Hydroactive gel. *American Journal of Perinatology, 21*, 409–414.

Lin, R. L., Tinkle, L. L., & Janniger, C. K. (2005). Skin care of the healthy newborn. *Cutis, 75*, 25–30.

Linder, N., Davidovitch, N., Reichman, B., Kuint, J., Lubin, D., Meyerovitch, J., ... Sack, J. (1997). Topical iodine-containing antiseptics and subclinical hypothyroidism in preterm infants. *Journal of Pediatrics, 131*, 434–439.

Linder, N., Prince, S., Barzilai, A., Keller, N., Klinger, G., Shalit, I., ... Sirota, L. (2004). Disinfection with 10% povidone-iodine versus 0.5% chlorhexidine gluconate in 70% isopropanol in the neonatal intensive care unit. *Acta Paediatrica 93*, 205–210.

Lineaweaver, W., Howard, R., Soucy, D., McMorris, S., Freeman, J., Crain, C., ... Rumley, T. (1985). Topical antimicrobial toxicity. *Archives of Surgery, 120*, 267–270.

Loring, C., Gregory, K., Gargan, B., Leblanc, V., Lundgren, D., Reilly, J., ... Zaya, C. (2012). Tub bathing improves thermoregulation of the late preterm infant. *Journal of Obstetric, Gynecologic, and Neonatal Nursing, 41*, 171–179. doi:10.1111/j.1552-6909.2011.01332.x

Lucky, A. W. (2008). Transient benign cutaneous lesions in the newborn. In L. A. Eichenfield, I. J. Frieden, & N. B. Esterly (Eds.), *Textbook of neonatal dermatology* (pp. 85–97). Philadelphia: W. B. Saunders.

Lund, C., Kuller, J., Lane, A., Lott, J., & Raines, D. (1999). Neonatal skin care: The scientific basis for practice. *Journal of Obstetric, Gynecologic, and Neonatal Nursing, 28*, 241–254.

Lund, C., & Tucker, J. (2003). Adhesion and newborn skin. In S. B. Hoath & H. I. Maibach (Eds.), *Neonatal skin: Structure and function* (2nd ed., pp. 269–291). New York: Marcel Dekker, Inc.

Lund, C. H., & Kuller, J. M. (2007). Integumentary system. In C. Kenner & J. W. Lott (Eds.), *Comprehensive neonatal care: An interdisciplinary approach* (4th ed., pp. 65–91). St. Louis, MO: Saunders Elsevier.

Lund, C. H., Kuller, J. M., Lane, A. T., Lott, J. W., Raines, D. A., & Thomas, K. K. (2001). Neonatal skin care: Evaluation of the AWHONN/NANN research-based practice project on knowledge and skin care practices. *Journal of Obstetric, Gynecologic, and Neonatal Nursing, 30*, 30–40.

Lund, C. H., Nonato, L. B., Kuller, J. M., Franck, L. S., Cullander, C., & Durand, D. J. (1997). Disruption of barrier function in neonatal skin associated with adhesive removal. *Journal of Pediatrics, 131,* 367–372.

Lund, C. H., & Osborne, J. W. (2004). Validity and reliability of the Neonatal Skin Condition Score. *Journal of Obstetric, Gynecologic, and Neonatal Nursing, 33,* 320–327.

Lund, C. H., Osborne, J. W., Kuller, J. M., Lane, A. T., Lott, J. W., & Raines, D. A. (2001). Neonatal skin care: Clinical outcomes of the AWHONN/NANN evidence-based clinical practice guideline. *Journal of Obstetric, Gynecologic, and Neonatal Nursing, 30,* 41–51.

Lundov, M. D., Moesby, L., Zachariae, C., & Johansen, J. D. (2009). Contamination versus preservation of cosmetics: A review on legislation, usage, infections, and contact allergy. *Contact Dermatitis, 60,* 70–78. doi:10.1111/j.1600-0536.2008.01501.x

Maayan-Metzger, A., Yosipovitch, G., Hadad, E., & Sirota, L. (2001). Transepidermal water loss and skin hydration in preterm infants during phototherapy. *American Journal of Perinatology, 18,* 393–396.

Maayan-Metzger, A., Yosipovitch, G., Hadad, E., & Sirota, L. (2004). Effect of radiant warmer on transepidermal water loss (TEWL) and skin hydration in preterm infants. *Journal of Perinatology, 24,* 372–375.

Maki, D. G., Ringer, M., & Alvarado, C. J. (1991). Prospective randomised trial of povidone-iodine, alcohol, and chlorhexidine for prevention of infection associated with central venous and arterial catheters. *Lancet, 338,* 339–343.

Malathi, I., Millar, M. R., Leeming, J. P., Hedges, A., & Marlow, N. (1993). Skin disinfection in preterm infants. *Archives of Disease in Childhood, 69,* 312–316.

Malloy, M. B., & Perez-Woods, R. C. (1991). Neonatal skin care: Prevention of skin breakdown. *Pediatric Nursing, 17,* 41–48.

Mancini, A. J. (2004). Skin. *Pediatrics, 113* (4 Suppl),1114-9.

Mancini, A. J., Sookdeo-Drost, S., Madison, K. C., Smoller, B. R., & Lane, A. T. (1994). Semipermeable dressings improve epidermal barrier function in premature infants. *Pediatric Research, 36,* 306–314.

Mannan, K., Chow, P., Lissauer, T., & Godambe, S. (2007). Mistaken identity of skin cleansing solution leading to extensive chemical burns in an extremely preterm infant. *Acta Paediatrica, 96,* 1536–1537. doi:10.1111/j.1651-2227.2007.00376.x

Marek, K. (1995). *Manual to develop guidelines.* ANA Committee on Nursing Practice Standards & Guidelines. Washington, DC: American Nurses Publishing, American Nurses Foundation/American Nurses Association.

Marks, J., Jr., Belsito, D., DeLeo, V., Fowler, J., Fransway, A., Maibach, H., … Taylor, J. (1995). North American Contact Dermatitis Group standard tray patch test results. *American Journal of Contact Dermatitis, 6,* 160–165.

Marlowe, L., Mistry, R. D., Coffin, S., Leckerman, K. H., McGowan, K. L., Dai, D., … Zaoutis, T. (2010). Blood culture contamination rates after skin antisepsis with chlorhexidine gluconate versus povidone-iodine in a pediatric emergency department. *Infection Control and Hospital Epidemiology, 31,* 171–176. doi:10.1086/650201

Marshall, A. (1997). Humidifying the environment for the premature neonate: Maintenance of a thermoneutral environment. *Journal of Neonatal Nursing, 3*, 32–36.

McCall, E. M., Alderice, F., Halliday, H. L., Jenkin, J. G., & Vohra, S. (2010). Interventions to prevent hypothermia in preterm and/or low birth weight infants. *Cochrane Database of Systematic Reviews*, Issue 3, Art. No.: CD004210. doi:10.1002/14651858.CD004210.pub4

McLane, K. M., Bookout, K., McCord, S., McCain, J., & Jefferson, L. S. (2004). The 2003 National Pediatric Pressure Ulcer and Skin Breakdown Prevalence Survey. *Journal of Wound, Ostomy and Continence Nursing, 31*, 168–178.

Meakins, S. (2006). The safety and toxicology of fragrances. In C. Sell (Ed.), *The chemistry of fragrances: From perfumer to consumer* (2nd ed.) (pp. 184-197). Cambridge, UK: The Royal Society of Chemistry.

Medves, J. M., & O'Brien, B. A. (1997). Cleaning solutions and bacterial colonization in promoting healing and separation of the umbilical cord in healthy newborns. *Canadian Journal of Public Health, 88*, 380–382.

Medves, J. M., & O'Brien, B. A. (2001). Does bathing newborns remove potentially harmful pathogens from the skin? *Birth, 28*, 161–165.

Medves, J. M., & O'Brien, B. A. (2004). The effect of bather and location of first bath on maintaining thermal stability in newborns. *Journal of Obstetric, Gynecologic, and Neonatal Nursing, 33*, 175–182.

Mendenhall, A. K., & Eichenfield, L. F. (2000). Back to basics: Caring for the newborn's skin. *Contemporary Pediatrics, 17*, 98–100, 103–104, 107–108.

Mermel, L. A. (2011). What is the predominant source of intravascular catheter infections? *Clinical Infectious Diseases, 52*, 211–212. doi:10.1093/cid/ciq108

Meyer, M. P., Payton, M. J., Salmon, A., Hutchinson, C., & de Klerk, A. (2001). A clinical comparison of radiant warmer and incubator care for preterm infants from birth to 1800 grams. *Pediatrics, 108*, 395–401.

Milstone, A. M., Passaretti, C. L., & Perl, T. M. (2008). Chlorhexidine: Expanding the armamentarium for infection control and prevention. *Clinical Infectious Diseases, 46*, 274–281. doi:10.1086/524736

Mitchell, I. M., Pollock, J. C., Jamieson, M. P., Fitzpatrick, K. C., & Logan, R. W. (1991). Transcutaneous iodine absorption in infants undergoing cardiac operation. *Annals of Thoracic Surgery, 52*, 1138–1140.

Moraille, R., Pickens, W., Visscher, M., Hoath, S. (2005). A novel role for vernix caseosa as a skin cleanser. *Biology of the Neonate, 87*, 8–14.

Morris, C., Emsley, P., Marland, E., Meuleneire, F., & White, R. (2009). Use of wound dressings with soft silicone adhesive technology. *Paediatric Nursing, 21*, 38–43.

Mullany, L. C., Darmstadt, G. L., Khatry, S. K., Katz, J., LeClerq, S. C., Shrestha, S., ... Tielsch, J. M. (2006). Topical applications of chlorhexidine to the umbilical cord for prevention of omphalitis and neonatal mortality in southern Nepal: A community-based, cluster-randomised trial. *Lancet, 367*, 910–918.

Mullany, L. C., Darmstadt, G. L., & Tielsch, J. M. (2003). Role of antimicrobial application to the umbilical cord in neonates to prevent bacterial colonization and infection: A review of the evidence. *Pediatric Infectious Disease Journal, 22*, 996–1002.

Mullany, L. C., Khatry, S. K., Sherchand, J. B., LeClerq, S. C., Darmstadt, G. L., Katz, J., ... Tielsch, J. M. (2008). A randomized controlled trial of the impact of chlorhexidine skin cleansing on bacterial colonization of hospital-born infants in Nepal. *Pediatric Infectious Disease Journal, 27*, 505–511. doi:10.1097/INF.0b013e31816791a2

Nako, Y., Harigaya, A., Tomomasa, T., Morikawa, A., Amada, M., Kijima, C., & Tsukagoshi, S. (2000). Effects of bathing immediately after birth on early neonatal adaptation and morbidity: A prospective randomized comparative study. *Pediatric International, 42*, 517–522.

Narendran, V., Wickett, R. R., Pickens, W. L., & Hoath, S. B. (2000). Interaction between pulmonary surfactant and vernix: A potential mechanism for induction of amniotic fluid turbidity. *Pediatric Research, 48*, 120–124. doi:10.1203/00006450-200007000-00021

Nicol, N. H. (2011). Efficacy and safety considerations in topical treatments for atopic dermatitis. *Pediatric Nursing, 37*, 295–301; quiz, 302.

Nield, L. S., & Kamat, D. (2007). Prevention, diagnosis, and management of diaper dermatitis. *Clinical Pediatrics, 46*, 480–486. doi:10.1177/0009922806292409

Nielsen, L. F., Blume, N., Romme, T., Samuelsen, P., Everland, H., Ifversen, P., & Karlsmark, T. (2005). Skin changes induced by a zinc oxide dressing compared with a hydrocolloid dressing in healthy individuals. *Skin Research and Technology, 11*, 140–151. doi:10.1111/j.1600-0846.2005.00105.x

Nikolovski, J., Stamatas, G. N., Kollias, N., & Wiegand, B. C. (2008). Barrier function and water-holding and transport properties of infant stratum corneum are different from adult and continue to develop through the first year of life. *Journal of Investigative Dermatology, 128*, 1728–1736.

Noonan, C., Quigley, S., & Curley, M. A. Q. (2011). Using the Braden Q Scale to predict pressure ulcer risk in pediatric patients. *Journal of Pediatric Nursing, 26*, 566–575. doi:10.1016/j.pedn.2010.07.006

Noonan, C., Quigley, S., & Curley, M. A. Q. (2006). Skin integrity in hospitalized infants and children: A prevalence survey. *Journal of Pediatric Nursing, 21*, 445–453. doi:10.1016/j.pedn.2006.07.002

Nopper, A. J., Horii, K. A., Sookdeo-Drost, S., Wang, T. H., Mancini, A. J., & Lane, A. T. (1996). Topical ointment therapy benefits premature infants. *Journal of Pediatrics, 128*, 660–669.

Odio, M., Streicher-Scott, J., & Hansen, R. C. (2001). Disposable baby wipes: Efficacy and skin mildness. *Dermatology Nursing, 13*, 107–121.

Ozon, A., Cetinkaya, S., Alikasifoglu, A., Gonc, E. N., Sen, Y., & Kandemir, N. (2007). Inappropriate use of potent topical glucocorticoids in infants. *Journal of Pediatric Endocrinology & Metabolism, 20*, 219–225.

Paller, A. S., Hawk, J. L. M., Honig, P., Giam, Y. C., Hoath, S., Mack, M. C., & Stamatas, G. N. (2011). New insights about infant and toddler skin: implications for sun protection. *Pediatrics, 128*(1), 92–102. doi:10.1542/peds.2010-1079

Parravicini, E., Fontana, C., Paterlini, G. L., Tagliabue, P., Rovelli, F., Leung, K., & Stark, R. I. (1996). Iodine, thyroid function, and very low birth weight infants. *Pediatrics, 98*, 730–734.

Perucca, R. (2010). Peripheral venous access devices. In M. Alexander, A. Corrigan, L. Gorski, J. Hankins, & R. Perucca R (Eds.), *Infusion nursing: An evidence-based approach* (3rd ed., pp. 456–479). St. Louis, MO: Saunders Elsevier.

Peters, K. L. (1998). Bathing premature infants: Physiological and behavioral consequences. *American Journal of Critical Care, 7*, 90–100.

Pettit, J. (2003). Assessment of the infant with a peripheral intravenous device. *Advances in Neonatal Care, 3*, 230–240.

Pezzati, M., Rossi, S., Tronchin, M., Dani, C., Filippi, L., & Rubattelli, F. (2003). Umbilical cord care in premature infants: The effect of two different cord-care regimens (salicylic sugar powder vs. chlorhexidine) on cord separation time and other outcomes. *Pediatrics, 112*, e275.

Polin, R. A., Denson, S., Brady, M. T., Committee on Fetus and Newborn, Committee on Infectious Diseases, American Academy of Pediatrics (2012). Strategies for prevention of health care-associated infections in the NICU. *Pediatrics, 129*, e1085–e1093. doi:10.1542/peds.2012-0145

Prizant, T. L., Lucky, A. W., Frieden, I. J., Burton, P. S., & Suarez, S. M. (1996). Spontaneous atrophic patches in extremely premature infants. *Archives of Dermatology, 132*, 671–674.

Quinn, D., Newton, N., & Piecuch, R. (2005). Effect of less frequent bathing on premature infant skin. *Journal of Obstetric, Gynecologic, and Neonatal Nursing, 34*, 741–746.

Rai, P., Lee, B.-M., Liu, T.-Y., Yuhui, Q., Krause, E., Marsman, D. S., & Felter, S. (2009). Safety evaluation of disposable baby diapers using principles of quantitative risk assessment. *Journal of Toxicology and Environmental Health, Part A, 72*, 1262–1271. doi:10.1080/15287390903212246

Ramasethu, J. (2004). Prevention and management of extravasation injuries in neonates. *NeoReviews, 5*, 491–497.

Reddy, K., Kogan, S., & Glick, S. A. (2011). Procedures and drugs in pediatric dermatology: Iatrogenic risks and situations of concern. *Clinics in Dermatology, 29*, 633–643. doi:10.1016/j.clindermatol.2011.08.028

Ressler-Maerlender, J., & Sorensen, R. E. (2005). Circumcision: An informed choice. *AWHONN Lifelines, 9*, 146–150.

Reynolds, P. R., Banerjee, S., & Meek, J. H. (2005). Alcohol burns in extremely low birthweight infants: Still occurring. *Archives of Disease in Childhood, Fetal and Neonatal Edition, 90*, F10.

Rissmann, R., Groenink, H. W. W., Gooris, G. S., Oudshoorn, M. H. M., Hennink, W. E., Ponec, M., & Bouwstra, J. A. (2008). Temperature-induced changes in structural and physicochemical properties of vernix caseosa. *Journal of Investigative Dermatology, 128*, 292–299. doi:10.1038/sj.jid.5701022

Rodeaver, G., (1989). Controversies in topical wound management. *Wounds, 1*, 19–27.

Rolstad, B. S., & Ovington, L. (2007). Principles of wound management. In R. A. Byrant & D. P. Nix (Eds.), *Acute & chronic wounds: Current management concepts* (3rd ed., pp. 391–426). St. Louis, MO: Mosby.

Russ, K. (2009). Health effects of personal care products: a review of the evidence. *Nursing for Women's Health, 13*(5), 392–401. doi:10.1111/j.1751-486X.2009.01457.x

Sankar, M. J., Paul, V. K., Kapil, A., Kalaivani, M., Agarwal, R., Darmstadt, G. L., & Deorari, A. K. (2009). Does skin cleansing with chlorhexidine affect skin condition, temperature and colonization in hospitalized preterm low birth weight infants? A randomized clinical trial. *Journal of Perinatology, 29,* 795–801. doi:10.1038/jp.2009.110

Sardesai, S. R., Kornacka, M. K., Walas, W., & Ramanathan, R. (2011). Iatrogenic skin injury in the neonatal intensive care unit. *Journal of Maternal-Fetal & Neonatal Medicine, 24,* 197–203. doi:10.3109/14767051003728245

Sarkar, R., Basu, S., Agrawal, R. K., & Gupta, P. (2010). Skin care for the newborn. *Indian Pediatrics, 47,* 593–598.

Sawatzky-Dicksson, D., & Bodnaryk, K. (2006). Neonatal intravenous extravasation injuries: Evaluation of a wound care protocol. *Neonatal Network, 25,* 13–19.

Scemons, D. J., & Elston, D. (Eds.). (2009). Principles of skin and wound care. In *Nurse to Nurse: Wound Care* (pp. 29–56) New York: McGraw-Hill Medical.

Scheinfeld, N. (2005). Diaper dermatitis. A review and brief survey of eruptions of the diaper area. *American Journal of Clinical Dermatology, 6,* 273–281.

Schick, J. B., & Milstein, J. M. (1981). Burn hazard of isopropyl alcohol in the neonate. *Pediatrics, 68,* 587–588.

Schindler, C. A., Mikhailov, T. A., Kuhn, E. M., Christopher, J., Conway, P., Ridling, D., ... Simpson, V. S. (2011). Protecting fragile skin: Nursing interventions to decrease development of pressure ulcers in pediatric intensive care. *American Journal of Critical Care, 20,* 26–34; quiz, 35. doi:10.4037/ajcc2011754

Schroeder, W. (2009). Understanding fragrance in personal care. *Cosmetics & Toiletries,124,* 36-44.

Scott, S. (2010). *Achieving consistent quality care: Using research to guide clinical practice* (2nd ed.). Washington, DC: Association of Women's Health, Obstetric and Neonatal Nurses.

Sedin, G., Hammarlund, K., Nilsson, G. E., Stromberg, B., & Oberg, P. A. (1985). Measurement of transepidermal water loss in newborn infants. *Clinics in Perinatology, 12,* 79–99.

Senarath, U., Fernando, D. N., & Rodrigo, I. (2007). Newborn care practices at home: Effect of a hospital-based intervention in Sri Lanka. *Journal of Tropical Pediatrics, 53,* 113–118. doi:10.1093/tropej/fml080

Shah, P. S., Ng, E., & Sinha, A. K. (2005). Heparin for prolonging peripheral intravenous catheter use in neonates. *Cochrane Database of Systematic Reviews,* Issue 4, Art. No.: CD002774. doi:10.1002/14651858.CD002774.pub2

Shin, H. T. (2005). Diaper dermatitis that does not quit. *Dermatologic Therapy, 18,* 124–135. doi:10.1111/j.1529-8019.2005.05013.x

Simona, R. (2012). A pediatric peripheral intravenous infiltration assessment tool. *Journal of Infusion Nursing, 35,* 243–248.

Simpson E., Berry, T., Brown, P., & Hanifin, J. (2010). A pilot study of emollient therapy for the primary prevention of atopic dermatitis. *Journal of the American Academy of Dermatology, 63*, 587–593.

Sinclair, L., Crisp, J., & Sinn, J. (2009). Variability in incubator humidity practices in the management of preterm infants. *Journal of Paediatrics and Child Health, 45*, 535–540. doi:10.1111/j.1440-1754.2009.01555.x

Smack, D. P., Harrington, A. C., Dunn, C., Howard, R. S., Szkutnik, A. J., Krivda, S. J., ... James, W.D. (1996). Infection and allergy incidence in ambulatory surgery patients using white petrolatum vs. bacitracin ointment. A randomized controlled trial. *Journal of the American Medical Association, 276*, 972–977.

Smerdely, P., Lim, A., Boyages, S. C, Waite, K., Wu, D., Roberts, V., ... Eastman, C. J. (1989). Topical iodine-containing antiseptics and neonatal hypothyroidism in very-low birthweight infants. *Lancet, 2*, 661–664.

Smith, W. J., & Jacob, S. E. (2009). The role of allergic contact dermatitis in diaper dermatitis. *Pediatric Dermatology, 26*, 369–370. doi:10.1111/j.1525-1470.2009.00934.x

Smoker, A. L. (2007). On top of cradle cap. *Journal of Family Health Care, 17*, 134–136.

Smolinski, K. N., Shah, S. S., Honig, P. J., & Yan, A. C. (2005). Neonatal cutaneous fungal infections. *Current Opinions in Pediatrics*,17, 486–493.

Soofi, S., Cousens, S., Imdad, A., Bhutto, N., Ali, N., & Bhutta, Z. A. (2012). Topical application of chlorhexidine to neonatal umbilical cords for prevention of omphalitis and neonatal mortality in a rural district of Pakistan: A community-based, cluster-randomised trial. *Lancet, 379*, 1029–1036. doi:10.1016/S0140-6736(11)61877-1

Soothill, J. S., Bravery, K., Ho, A., Macqueen, S., Collins, J., & Lock, P. (2009). A fall in bloodstream infections followed a change to 2% chlorhexidine in 70% isopropanol for catheter connection antisepsis: A pediatric single center before/after study on a hemopoietic stem cell transplant ward. *American Journal of Infection Control, 37*, 626–630. doi:10.1016/j.ajic.2009.03.014

Spraker, M. K., Gisoldi, E. M., Siegfried, E. C., Fling, J. A., de Espinosa, Z. D., Quiring, J. N., & Zangrillis, S. G. (2006). Topical miconazole nitrate ointment in the treatment of diaper dermatitis complicated by candidiasis. *Cutis, 77*, 113–120.

Spencer, S. P., Shields, B. J., & Smith, G. A. (2005). Childhood bathtub-related injuries: slip and fall prevalence and prevention. *Clinical Pediatrics, 44*, 311–318.

Stamatas, G., Nikolovski, J., Mack, M., & Kollias, N. (2011). Infant skin physiology and development during the first years of life: A review of recent findings based on in vivo studies. *International Journal of Cosmetic Science, 33*, 17–24. doi:10. 1111/j.146/j.1468-2494.2010.00611.x

Stamatas, G. N., Zerweck, C., Grove, G., & Martin, K. M. (2011). Documentation of impaired epidermal barrier in mild and moderate diaper dermatitis in vivo using noninvasive methods. *Pediatric Dermatology, 28*, 99–107. doi:10.1111/j.1525-1470.2011.01308.x

Stephen-Haynes, J. (2008). Skin integrity and silicone: Appeel "no-sting" medical adhesive remover. *British Journal of Nursing, 17*(12), 792–795.

Stokowski, L. (2006, Summer). Neonatal skin: Back to nature. *Midwifery Today, 78*, 34–35.

Stotts, N. A. (2007). Nutritional assessment and support. In R. A. Byrant & D. P. Nix (Eds.), *Acute & chronic wounds: Current management concepts* (3rd ed., pp. 149–160). St. Louis, MO: Mosby.

Suddaby, E. C., Barnett, S., & Facteau, L. (2005). Skin breakdown in acute care pediatrics. *Pediatric Nursing 31,* 132–148.

Suliman, A. K., Watts, H., Beiler, J., King, T. S., Khan, S., Carnuccio, M., & Paul, I. M. (2010). Triple dye plus rubbing alcohol versus triple dye alone for umbilical cord care. *Clinical Pediatrics, 49,* 45–48. doi:10.1177/0009922808329455

Tamma, P. D., Aucott, S. W., & Milstone, A. M. (2010). Chlorhexidine use in the neonatal intensive care unit: Results from a national survey. *Infection Control and Hospital Epidemiology, 31,* 846–849. doi:10.1086/655017

Tansirikongkol, A., Visscher, M. O., & Wickett, R. R. (2007). Water-handling properties of vernix caseosa and a synthetic analogue. *Journal of Cosmetic Science, 58,* 651–662.

Tapia-Rombo, C. A., Morales-Mora, M., & Alvarez-Vazquez, E. (2003). Variations of vital signs, skin color, behavior and oxygen saturation in premature neonates after sponge bathing. Possible complications. *Revista de Investigación Clínica, 55,* 438–443.

Taquino, L. T. (2000). Promoting wound healing in the neonatal setting: Process versus protocol. *Journal of Perinatal & Neonatal Nursing, 14,* 104–118.

Thigpen, J. L. (2007). Peripheral intravenous extravasation: Nursing procedure for initial treatment. *Neonatal Network, 26,* 379–384.

Thomas, S., Rowe, H., Keats, S., & Morgan, R. (1997 October). The management of extravasation injury in neonates. *World Wide Wounds.* Retrieved from http://www.worldwidewounds.com/1997/october/Neonates/NeonatePaper.html

Tollin, M., Bersson, G., Kai-Larsen, Y., Lengqvist, J., Sjovall, J., Griffiths, W., … Agerberth, B. (2005). Vernix caseosa as a multi-component defence system based on polypeptides, lipids and their interactions. *Cellular and Molecular Life Science, 62,* 2390–2399.

Topper, W. H., & Stewart, T. P. (1984). Thermal support for the very-low-birth-weight infant: Role of supplemental conductive heat. *Journal of Pediatrics, 105,* 810–814.

Tyebkhan, G. (2002). Skin cleansing in neonates and infants—basics of cleansers. *Indian Journal of Pediatrics, 69,* 767–769.

Turnbaugh, P., Ley, R., Hamady, M., Fraser-Liggett, C., Knight, R., & Gordon, J. (2007). The human microbiome project. *Nature, 449,* 804–810.

United States Food & Drug Administration. (2012). *2% chlorhexidine gluconate (CHG) cloth. Detailed view: Safety labeling changes approved by FDA Center for Drug Evaluation and Research (CDER)—May 2012.* Retrieved from http://www.fda.gov/Safety/MedWatch/SafetyInformation/Safety-RelatedDrugLabelingChanges/ucm307387.htm

United States Food and Drug Administration (2009). Cosmetics: Laws and regulations. Retrieved from http://www.fda.gov/Cosmetics/GuidanceComplianceRegulatoryInformation/ActsRulesRegulations/default.htm

United States Preventive Services Task Force. (1996). *Guide to clinical preventive services (2nd ed.)*. Baltimore: Williams & Wilkins.

Varda, K. E., & Behnke, R. S. (2000). The effect of timing of initial bath on newborn's temperature. *Journal of Obstetric, Gynecologic, and Neonatal Nursing, 29*, 27–32.

Vernon, H. J., Lane, A. T., Wischerath, L. J., Davis, J. M., & Menegus, M. A. (1990). Semipermeable dressing and transepidermal water loss in premature infants. *Pediatrics, 86*, 357–362.

Varughese M & Koh T. (2001). Successful Use of Topical Nitroglycerine in Ischemia Associated with Umbilical Arterial Line in a Neonate, 2001. *Journal of Perinatology, 21*, 556-558.

Vender, R. B. (2003). Adverse reactions to herbal therapy in dermatology. *Skin therapy letter, 8*(3), 5–8.

Visscher, M., Chatterjee, R., Ebel, J., LaRuffa, A., & Hoath, S. (2002). Biomedical assessment and instrumental evaluation of healthy infant skin. *Pediatric Dermatology, 19*, 473–482.

Visscher, M., de Castro, M. V., Combs, L., Perkins, L., Winer, J., Schwegman, N., & Bondurant, P. (2009). Effect of chlorhexidine gluconate on the skin integrity at PICC line sites. *Journal of Perinatology, 29*, 802–807. doi:10.1038/jp.2009.116

Visscher, M., Narendran, V., Pickens, W., LaRuffa, A., Meinzen-Derr, J., Allen, K., & Hoath, S. B. (2005). Vernix caseosa in neonatal adaptation. *Journal of Perinatology, 25*, 440–446.

Visscher, M., Odio, M., Taylor, T., White, T., Sargent, S., Sluder, L., ... Bondurant, P. (2009). Skin care in the NICU patient: Effects of wipes versus cloth and water on stratum corneum integrity. *Neonatology, 96*, 226–234. doi:10.1159/000215593

Visscher, M. O., Barai, N., LaRuffa, A. A., Pickens, W. L., Narendran, V., & Hoath, S. B. (2011). Epidermal barrier treatments based on vernix caseosa. *Skin Pharmacology and Physiology, 24*, 322–329. doi:10.1159/000328744

Visscher, M. O., Chatterjee, R., Munson, K. A., Bare, D. E., & Hoath, S. B. (2000). Changes in diapered and nondiapered infant skin over the first month of life. *Pediatric Dermatology, 17*, 45–51.

Vohra, S., Frent, G., Campbell, V., Abbott, M., & Whyte, R. (1999). Effects of polyethylene occlusive skin wrapping on heat loss in very low birth weight infants at delivery: A randomized trial. *Journal of Pediatrics, 134*, 547–551.

Vohra, S., Roberts, R. S., Zhang, B., Janes, M., & Schmidt, B. (2004). Heat loss prevention (HeLP) in the delivery room: A randomized controlled trial of polyethylene occlusive skin wrapping in very preterm infants. *Journal of Pediatrics, 145*, 720–722.

Vural, G., & Sezer, K. (2006). Umbilical cord care: A pilot study comparing topical human milk, povidone-iodine and dry care. *Journal of Obstetric, Gynecologic, and Neonatal Nursing, 35*, 123–128.

Wada, M., Kusuda, S., Takahashi, N., & Nishida, H. (2008). Fluid and electrolyte balance in extremely preterm infants <24 weeks of gestation in the first week of life. *Pediatrics International, 50*, 331–336. doi:10.1111/j.1442-200X.2008.02577.x

Wananukul, S., & Praisuwanna, P. (2002). Clear topical ointment decreases transepidermal water loss in jaundiced preterm infants receiving phototherapy. *Journal of the Medical Association of Thailand, 85,* 102–106.

Wananukul, S., Praisuwanna, P., & Kesorncam, K. (2001). Effects of clear topical ointment on transepidermal water loss in jaundiced preterm infants receiving phototherapy. *Journal of the Medical Association of Thailand, 84,* 837–841.

Watson, J. (2006). Community-associated methicillin-resistant *Staphylococcus aureus* infection among healthy newborns—Chicago and Los Angeles County, 2004. *MMWR: Morbidity & Mortality Weekly Report, 3,* 329.

Weber, B., Speer, M., Swartz, D., Rupp, S., O'Linn, W., & Stone, K. (1987). Irritation and stripping effects of adhesive tapes on skin layers of coronary bypass graft patients. *Heart & Lung, 16,* 567–572.

Webster, J., & McCosker, H. (1994). Cardiac monitoring in the neonatal intensive care unit: An evaluation of electrodes. *Neonatal Network, 13,* 51–54.

Weinstein, S. (2007). Pediatric intravenous therapy. In S. M. Weinstein. *Plumer's Principles & Practice of Intravenous Therapy* (8th ed., p. 647). Philadelphia: Lippincott Williams & Wilkins.

Weitz, N. A. (2013). Chlorhexidine gluconate–impregnated central access catheter dressings as a cause of erosive contact dermatitis: A report of 7 cases. *JAMA Dermatology, 149,* 195. doi:10.1001/jamadermatol.2013.903

White, M. C., Kalus, J. S., Caron, M. F., & Suski, K. (2003). Cholestyramine ointment used on an infant for severe buttocks rash resistant to standard therapeutic modalities. *Journal of Pharmacy Technology, 19,* 11–13.

Wilson, J. R., Mills, J. G., Prather, I. D., & Dimitrijevich, S. D. (2005). A toxicity index of skin and wound cleansers used on in vitro fibroblasts and keratinocytes. *Advances in Skin & Wound Care, 18,* 373–378.

Witt, C. (2004). *Neonatal dermatology.* In M. Verklan & M. Walden (Eds.), *Core curriculum for neonatal intensive care nursing* (pp. 893–912). St. Louis, MO: Elsevier Saunders Publishers.

Woods, A. G., & Cederholm, C. K. (2012). Subcutaneous fat necrosis and whole-body cooling therapy for neonatal encephalopathy. *Advances in Neonatal Care, 12,* 345–348. doi:10.1097/ANC.0b013e3182613bff

Woolf, A. D. (2003). Herbal remedies and children: Do they really work? Are they harmful? *Pediatrics, 112,* 240-246.

Woolf, S. H. (1990). *Interim manual for clinical practice guideline development.* Washington, DC: Agency for Health Care Policy and Research.

Woolf, S. H. (1992). Practice guidelines, a new reality in medicine: II. Methods of developing guidelines. *Archives of Internal Medicine, 152,* 946–952.

World Health Organization. (2006). *Pregnancy, childbirth, postpartum and newborn care: A guide for essential practice.* Geneva, Switzerland: Author.

Yoshio, H., Lagercrantz, H., Gudmundsson, G., & Agerbeth, B. (2004). First line of defense in early human life. *Seminars in Perinatology, 28,* 304–311.

Youssef, W., Wickett, R., & Hoath, S. (2001). Surface free energy characterization of vernix caseosa: Potential role in waterproofing the newborn infant. *Skin Research and Technology, 7*, 10–17.

Yosipovitch, G., Maayan-Metzger, A., Merlob, P. P., & Sirota, L. (2000). Skin barrier properties in different body areas in neonates. *Pediatrics, 106*, 105–108.

Zilmer R., Agren, M. S., Gottrup, F., & Karlsmark, T. (2006) Biophysical effects of removal of adhesive dressings on peri-ulcer skin. *Journal of Wound Care, 15,* 187–191.

Zupan, J., Garner, P., & Omari, A. A. A. (2004). Topical umbilical cord care at birth. *Cochrane Database of Systematic Reviews*, Issue 3. Art. No.: CD001057. doi:10.1002/14651858.CD001057

APPENDIX A

AWHONN Neonatal Skin Condition Score Tool

AWHONN Neonatal Skin Condition Score (NSCS)

Dryness

1 = Normal, no sign of dry skin

2 = Dry skin, visible scaling

3 = Very dry skin, cracking/fissures

Erythema

1 = No evidence of erythema

2 = Visible erythema, <50% body surface

3 = Visible erythema, ≥50% body surface

Breakdown

1 = None evident

2 = Small, localized areas

3 = Extensive

Note: perfect score = 3, worst score = 9.

This scoring system, developed for the AWHONN/NANN Neonatal Skin Care Research-Based Practice Project (RBP4), was adapted from a visual scoring system used in a previous study (Lane & Drost, 1993). This tool can facilitate assessment of neonatal skin condition.

Copyright 2007. Association of Women's Health, Obstetric and Neonatal Nurses. This skin assessment tool may be duplicated for use in the clinical setting. It is understood that institutions may have different resources, and the states or provinces where the institutions are located may promulgate different regulations. This tool does not define a standard of care, nor is it intended to dictate an exclusive course of management. This tool presents general methods and techniques of practice that are currently accepted and used by recognized authorities.

APPENDIX B

Suggested Perineal Skin Care Guidelines for Diapered/Incontinent Patients

© The Children's Hospital of Philadelphia. Adapted with Permission.

Skin Assessment	• Intact skin • No erythema	• Intact skin • High risk for skin breakdown due to causticity of stool (short gut, post pull through or ostomy closure) • With or without erythema	• Intact skin • Erythema • No *Candida***	• Intact skin • Erythema, satellite lesions typically on thighs, perineum • Evidence of *Candida***	• Denuded skin* • No *Candida***	• Denuded skin* • Evidence of *Candida***†
Goal of Treatment	Prevent skin breakdown	Prevent skin breakdown; Provide barrier	Prevent skin breakdown; Provide barrier	Treat *Candida*	Prevent further skin breakdown; Provide barrier	Prevent further skin breakdown; Provide barrier
No-Sting Barrier film may be applied prior to application of any of the below products (in patients > 28 days old)						
Treatment	Petrolatum	Zinc oxide barrier cream **OR** Alcohol-free, pectin-based paste, covered with petrolatum	Zinc oxide barrier cream	Antifungal topical treatment	Pectin powder then zinc oxide barrier cream **OR** Pectin powder then alcohol-free, pectin-based paste then petrolatum **OR** One of above plus crusting technique	Antifungal ointment or cream then zinc oxide barrier cream **OR** Antifungal powder and alcohol-free skin protectant crusting technique then alcohol-free, pectin-based paste then petrolatum
Application Instructions	Apply a thick layer of petrolatum over the entire area to be protected (think "icing on a cake").	Apply a thick layer of zinc oxide-based cream (think "icing on a cake"). **OR** **For alcohol-free, pectin-based paste:** • "Press" into place vs. "spreading." • Apply a thick layer of petrolatum on top of pectin product, to prevent pectin product from sticking to diaper. **With each diaper change:** • Only remove stool, try to leave pectin product in place. • If skin showing, replace pectin product as needed, re-apply petrolatum.	Apply a thick layer of zinc oxide-based cream (think "icing on a cake").	Apply antifungal ointment; if no improvement in 24-48 hours, consider using a different antifungal preparation.	Apply a thin layer of pectin powder to denuded areas. Brush off excess. Powder will stick to the open skin. Then apply thick layer of zinc oxide barrier cream or alcohol-free, pectin-based paste on top of pectin powder. **For alcohol-free, pectin-based paste:** • Press into place vs. spreading. • Apply thick layer of petrolatum over pectin product to prevent pectin from sticking to diaper. **With each diaper change:** • Only remove stool, try to leave pectin product in place. • Skin showing: replace pectin product prn, re-apply petrolatum. **Crusting Technique:** Pectin powder, then seal with alcohol-free skin protectant. Repeat this step, then layer alcohol-free, pectin based paste or zinc oxide cream.	Apply antifungal ointment or cream, followed by zinc oxide barrier cream. **OR** **Crusting Technique:** Apply a thin layer of antifungal powder to denuded areas. Brush off excess. Then apply thick layer alcohol-free, pectin-based paste or zinc oxide barrier cream on top of antifungal powder layer.

*Denuded Skin: Skin with moist, open, oozing ulcerations.
***Candida* infection: Beefy red skin with oval/ dotty lesions scattered at edges (satellite lesions), usually involves skin folds, skin may or may not be denuded.
NOTE: These products promote moist wound healing, therefore do not leave diaper open to air or have air/oxygen blowing on diaper area
† Source: ©Douglas Hoffman, MD, Dermatlas. http://www.dermatlas.org

APPENDIX C

Product Selection Considerations

This document provides general information that clinicians may find helpful when making decisions or counseling patients about selection of topical skin care products for neonates. It is meant to serve as a quick reference. This document is not all-inclusive and is not intended to be used as a substitute for the evidence-based guideline. Clinicians should consult this evidence-based guideline for recommendations about cleansers, and other reliable sources of information to determine which products and product categories are appropriate and safe for their individual patient's needs.

General Considerations:

- Read product labels. This is important for both clinicians and consumers. By doing so, clinicians can enhance their awareness of product formulations and can help parents be better informed about ingredients that may have the potential to cause alterations in skin integrity.
- Be aware that parents may have culturally based needs and desires for skin care and products for their newborn babies.
- Communicate with families based on their concerns and questions about skin care products.
- Assess parents' personal and family histories to identify risks for barrier dysfunction, e.g., history of skin sensitivity, dermatitis or other skin problems.
- Recommend that the amount of product applied on infants should be limited to only those products that are necessary. Limiting the use of products will reduce the risk of contact sensitization.
- Select products or advise families that they should select products that ideally have been safety-tested on neonates or infants. Products containing preservatives should have a demonstrated safety and tolerability in newborns. Mild products are preferable.
- Be aware of and be prepared to discuss with families general information about how newborn skin care products are regulated. For example, the U.S. Food and Drug Administration (FDA) regulate cosmetics to some degree according to the Federal Food, Drug, and Cosmetic Act and, for products marketed on a retail basis to consumers, the Fair Packaging and Labeling Act. Cosmetics include baby care products, such as baby shampoos, lotions, oils, powders and other baby care products (FDA, 2013). The regulation of cosmetics is a complex process that is shared by different agencies (Lundov et al., 2009), and manufacturers are primarily responsible for ensuring the safety of their products (Russ, 2009).
- Consult professional associations and other federal resources. A listing of some of these resources is provided at the end of this document.

Selected Product Categories:

Cleansers

The role of cleansers is to emulsify oil, dirt, and microorganisms on the skin surface so they can be easily removed with water.

- Ideally, cleansers should not cause skin irritation, disrupt the normal pH of the skin surface, or cause stinging or irritation of the eyes.
- Select mild liquid cleansers or cleansing bars that have a neutral or mildly acidic pH (pH 5.5-7.0) or those that have been shown to have minimal impact on the baby's skin surface pH.
- Choose cleansers with preservatives that have demonstrated safety and tolerability for newborns. Preservatives are usually needed to prevent the overgrowth of microorganisms that may occur with normal use, but preservatives may result in skin irritation or contact dermatitis.

Fragrances

- Fragrances are added to many products for customer appeal. According to the USFDA, any ingredient added solely to impart scent should be listed as "fragrance" or "parfum" on the product label. Products may be labeled as "fragrance free" if the scent-imparting ingredient is added for another purpose, e.g., masking the odor of the product or preserving the product. Unscented means that a product has been formulated to have no scent. Unscented products may still contain a fragrance if it is added to mask the odor of the product (Bridges, 2002).

- Fragrances are typically classified into 3 groups (Schroeder 2009): essential oils, which are derived from plants; natural fragrances, which are derived from a natural source; and synthetic fragrances, which are man-made. Some synthetic fragrances may be identical to molecules derived from a natural source (Schroeder, 2009). Natural fragrances are not always considered to be safer than synthetic fragrances, because some ingredients such as natural essential oils may be allergens or irritants (Meakens, 2006).

Organic, Natural and Herbal Products

- There is limited data available about many natural and organic products, and definitions of these categories of products may also vary. Although many herbal therapy products may be safe for adult use, caution is recommended for use in newborns since some of these products have not been tested on neonates (Vender, 2003; Woolf, 2003).
- Allergic contact dermatitis, or eczema, is the most common skin condition resulting from the use of herbal therapies. Some of the herbs known for causing this reaction include aloe, arnica, bromelain, calendula, chamomile, goldenseal, tea tree oil and yarrow (Vender, 2003).

Sunscreens

A sunscreen is a compound that reflects, absorbs or scatters the harmful spectrum of UV light. There is little data about the safety and efficacy of sunscreen in children younger than 6 months of age. Therefore, safe practice for neonates and infants is generally to avoid sun exposure, followed by use of appropriate protective clothing along with application of zinc-oxide-containing sunscreens to cover areas that are uncovered, e.g., the face and hands (Bree & Siegfried, 2008). General considerations for neonatal sunscreen use include but are not limited to the following:

- If sun exposure cannot be completely avoided, the newborn should be dressed in lightweight long pants, long-sleeved shirts, and hats with brims that ideally shade the neck to prevent sunburn. Newborns should be kept in shaded areas when outside, and avoid sun exposure during midday (AAP, 2009; Aulbert, 2009; Dadlani & Orlow, 2008; Paller, 2011).
- When necessary, small amounts of sunscreen with a Sun Protection Factor (SPF) of 15 can be applied to small areas of exposed skin (Paller, 2011).

Provider and Consumer Resources:

The following is a list of professional organizations that clinicians and consumers can consult to retrieve additional information about neonatal and pediatric skin care products and safety profiles:

- American Academy of Allergy, Asthma and Immunology http://www.aaaai.org/home.aspx
- American Academy of Dermatology http://www.aad.org
- American Academy of Pediatrics http://www.healthychildren.org
- Association of Women's Health, Obstetric and Neonatal Nurses http://www.awhonn.org
- Federal Trade Commission Consumer Protection Agency http://www.ftc.gov/bcp/consumer.shtm
- Centers for Disease Control and Prevention http://www.cdc.gov/
- Food and Drug Administration (http://www.fda.gov/Cosmetics)
- Wound, Ostomy and Continence Nurses Society http://www.wocn.org/

Clinicians and consumers can find valuable information about how to assess the quality of consumer websites by consulting university websites designed for this purpose. Examples include, but are not limited to:

- Cornell University: http://olinuris.library.cornell.edu/ref/research/webeval.html
- University of Maryland: http://www.lib.umd.edu/ues/guides/evaluating-web
- The Johns Hopkins University: http://guides.library.jhu.edu/evaluatinginformation

APPENDIX D

Continuing Nursing Education Credit Information

NEONATAL SKIN CARE: EVIDENCE-BASED CLINICAL PRACTICE GUIDELINE, 3RD EDITION

2.8 contact hours of CNE credit for this program may be earned until December 31, 2015.
[These contact hours are calculated based on a 60-minute hour.]

Instructions

- To obtain contact hours you must purchase CNE in the AWHONN Store and complete an online post-test and feedback form.
- To purchase CNE, visit the AWHONN Store at www.awhonn.org/store and purchase the CNE Companion for Neonatal Skin Care, Evidence-Based Clinical Practice Guideline, 3rd Edition, item #CNE-ENSC-3. The price is $15 for members and $25 for non-members.
- After purchasing CNE visit www.awhonn.org/CNE to complete the online post-test and feedback form. Make sure you have your order number ready. Your order number can be found in the receipt that was emailed after purchase.
- Questions regarding this program or the process of applying for CNE credit should be directed to (800) 673-8499 or (800) 245-0231 from Canada, or via email at cne@awhonn.org.

Association of Women's Health, Obstetric and Neonatal Nurses is accredited as a provider of continuing nursing education by the American Nurses Credentialing Center's Commission on Accreditation.

AWHONN is approved by the California Board of Registered Nursing, Provider #CEP580.

Accredited status does not imply endorsement by AWHONN or the American Nurses Credentialing Center of any commercial products displayed or discussed in conjunction with educational activities.

AWHONN has been recognized as ANCC Premier Program Provider for Innovation in Continuing Nurse Education.